# Reboot Your Nervous System

## The Quantum Needle Trilogy:
## Book 1

## Medical Meditations

Visit www.RebootYourNervousSystem.com
to listen to audio meditations

**Follow on Instagram**

**Reboot Website**

**Audio**

# Dedication

To my immediate family
Terry and Olivia

To patients
who aspire to heal

To my fellow practitioners
who endeavor to help those in need

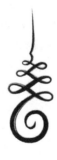

# Acknowledgements

Many people supported me and this project. I'm thankful to: Peter Taylor for sharing 50 years of friendship and 6 years of this research, Manya Bean for living the work, Kareen Novak for doing the work, Marina Bean for her insight, the Wisotsky clan for their hearts and skills, and Bobby Riley for his keen understanding. Our many discussions helped immensely. I'm so grateful to my wife Terry Wilson, and daughter, Olivia, who helped me stay the course!

I love my team at Pacific Center of Health, my clinical home. Serving patients is the ultimate honor, but being at the helm of this esteemed group of healers is my second highest achievement. I deeply appreciate my teachers at the Barral Institute: my first teacher Dee Ahern in 1996, Leilani Lee for mentoring me for decades, and Jean Anne Zollars who recruited me to step up and teach. Your generosity empowered me to grow! I have also been blessed with talented musical friends, who helped me hear beauty and CoCreate harmony.

To my editors, Rani Kronick and Amy Delue, I *literally* couldn't have done this without you! To my esteemed webmaster Julie Silva, I owe you big time! Robin Ross-Wisotsky added artistry to the cover design, and she also spruced up many images in the book. Sak Joker from Fiverr also lent his skillset to my logo and graphics.

My most sincere gratitude goes to my elder brother, **Justin Bean**, who has contributed so much creative energy. He is responsible for the art and images that bring this text to life. His artful work utilizes all of his attributes: his eye, his imagination, his pen, his CrAIyon, his hands, and his humor.

# Table of Contents

# Foreword

Adrian and I have been friends since we went to preschool together in Atlantic City, New Jersey. That was before there were casinos there. I have a unique perspective on his career as an acupuncturist, manual therapist, and energy healer. I have witnessed his practice grow and evolve, as he has grown and evolved in his practice. I have received treatments, herbs, needles, and energetic adjustments, periodically over the past twenty-five years and although the treatments have evolved, the essence has remained steady. That essence is the Reboot.

As Adrian became a master healer in San Diego, California, I studied meditation under a Korean Zen master in Toronto, Canada and became a Zen master myself. The aim of Zen practice is to learn to live peacefully with your own ego, which is mostly done by sitting in meditation, watching thoughts arise and then letting them go. The aim of the Reboot is similar in that it is another path to help us put down our egos and enter an extra relaxed and ultimately healing state of mind. It was funny to me as an experienced meditator to go through a treatment where Adrian instructed me to just let myself go, relax my face, drop my mask. It was funny because that was what I had been trying to do all along through hours and hours of focused meditation. Why not just do it? Why not?

It is fitting that Adrian would be a big part of my journey to dismantle my ego, because growing up together, we created our egos in consultation with each other and strengthened them by smashing them into each other. We developed these egos in the 1980's, an era famed for its over-the-top egocentricity. It was at that time that Adrian introduced me to my first paradigm shift.

After reading Carlos Castanada's books of shaman apprenticeship in Mexico, Adrian convinced me that the books were about something real.

In my limited, egotistical, teenaged understanding, I knew all that stuff, including Zen and acupuncture, was superstitious nonsense. Adrian knew better. Using a technique from the book, he was able to awaken into a lucid dream. Every night I tried to do the same, partly because it would be cool, and partly because Adrian could do it and my ego wanted to match his skills. I never become a lucid dreamer, but I learned that more is possible than I ever thought possible.

The second time Adrian helped me wrap my head around a new paradigm was much later in our lives. I was well into my Zen practice, which had taught me way more about how much I didn't know, but I still thought I knew things. Adrian was talking passionately about Oneness, a natural order to the universe (or multiverse as he prefers). I had always considered the idea of any kind of God a hard pill to swallow. I was fine with people like the Buddha, who discovered and taught techniques to transcend suffering, but was not himself a god. However, as Adrian described this intelligence happening in our cells and in the plants and animals all around us, I realized that my quiet atheism was just more of me thinking I knew things that I didn't really know. So maybe there's a God. Go figure.

God is immaterial to the work of Rebooting. It is just another example of how our egos build themselves around beliefs that may or may not be helpful or accurate. Whether we believe it or not, our bodies know how to get things done intelligently. The intelligence we are so proud of, the one that makes us think we are smarter or dumber than each other, often gets in the way of our health. Our egos and personal intelligence can work against us by systematically resisting the relaxation that is so good for us. The Reboot lets us address that head on as Adrian teaches us the techniques we need to heal ourselves.

The work of the Reboot, the work of Zen, and the work of life is to find some comfort in an often-uncomfortable body. Our bodies are prone to all sorts of physical and mental discomforts, and over the years those discomforts have a way of integrating themselves into our systems. They become such a part of us that we don't imagine that there could be another way. Good news, you can always Reboot. Lie down, relax, breathe, and let yourself go. I have been lucky throughout my life to have such a talented healer and meta philosopher as my friend. You are lucky to have Adrian's years of experience, insight and compassion available to you too. Please enjoy it.

In gratitude,

Peter Taylor

Zen Master in the Chogye Order of Korean Buddhism

Check out Peter's Zen books series: **amazon.com/author/zenpeter**

His blog: **zenmister.substack.com**

His family farm: **TaylorsFarm.org**

**Peter's Blog**

# Intro to Self-Healing:

## Restoring Feedback to Body & Mind

My experience with self-healing began as a 20-year-old college student studying math and physics when I became quite ill with Lyme disease. I took antibiotics which helped immensely at first, but six months later I had troubling and worsening symptoms. I saw many doctors but nothing worked, so I felt discouraged and defeated by my deteriorating condition. When confronted with the harsh reality of chronic illness, I initially retreated into self-pity and the victim mindset of "woe is me."

After a few months I realized this victim persona didn't define me. I was physically ill and simultaneously stressed about being sick, so I was trapped in 2 vicious cycles involving both body and mind. My physical symptoms made me depressed, and my doubts weakened my body. When I recognized this pattern as a crashed loop that creates suffering, I vowed to break the cycle by any means necessary. I saw that my disease had inertia, which implies it would tend to continue unless acted upon by an outside force. The impulse to do whatever it takes activated my will, an internal force that can change the trajectory of a person's life. I applied my attention diligently using yoga, breathing, diet, herbs, and meditation. I slowly regained vitality and learned many lessons, mostly the hard way. One day, as if struck by lightning, I realized I could provide others with the help I needed when I was young and sick, inspiring me to train in the healing arts.

I became an acupuncturist and herbalist. I am also a manual therapist specializing in anatomically precise cranial osteopathy and Visceral Manipulation, a method to treat organs that was developed by JeanPierre Barral. We train our hands to palpate the various tissues including fascia, organs, the spine, and nerves.  We also treat bones, joints, and even arteries. The method, called induction, is to feel into the tissue and activate the mechanoreceptors, which signals the brain to reassess the wounded area. I teach for the Barral Institute and I have trained many acupuncturists, bodyworkers, physical therapists, and MDs.  In my clinical practice, I have had the opportunity to treat tens of thousands of patients and I have learned invaluable lessons from each one. I have taught many to meditate, deepen their yoga practice, and flow with Tai Chi. I will present simple tools borne out of my personal journey and my clinical experience to help you find your personal path to health and wellbeing.

Every living body is trying to survive and maintain its metabolism. Our cells perpetually harness the energy that keeps us alive. These tiny, biochemical machines produce our metabolic energy, the Qi that propels us onward.  Hooray for life giving cells! Healing is simply a byproduct of this natural process called life. Ultimately, all healing is self-healing, because the body repairs itself.  The cells do the work.

Healers don't heal the patient; we set up the conditions where the patient can self-heal. We *facilitate* the healing.  For example, putting a cast on a broken bone holds it steady, giving the cells an opportunity to repair the break. Injecting stem cells into damaged tissue allows *them* to rebuild the tissue. Cutting out a malignant tumor can save a person's life, but oddly that doesn't heal them. The mechanisms that built the cancerous cells aren't addressed when you remove a tumor. All of these treatments *alter the conditions* within the body for the better. The Reboot Meditation sets up the optimal conditions that empower your self-healing. It doesn't cut away tumors, but it dismantles destructive patterns that degrade you. The Reboot doesn't inject you with stem cells, but it activates your deep, intrinsic abilities to repair what has been damaged and remake yourself anew.

Like everything else, life and healing are governed by natural forces. As a modern acupuncturist I've been investigating the forces that produce and sustain life from an Eastern and Western perspective. My job is to help patients by researching how to harness the natural resources that can heal them. Qi is usually defined as *energy and breath*. While this might sound poetic or vague, energy and breath describes cellular respiration, the metabolism within our mitochondria that manufactures our energy. Breathing adds the oxygen which catalyses the biochemistry that produces the energy that animates us. Qi is our metabolic life-force. This metabolic Qi energy, acquired from breathing, animates the nervous system and becomes the electrical spark that keeps your heart beating. Qi is biochemical energy and it is also the electrical current coursing through your nerves, your brain and your acupuncture meridians. I'm a "Qi electrician," and I'll train you to access your electrical Qi and direct it toward self-healing. The Reboot Method combines the best of East and West: meditative inquiry and scientific discovery.

Science transformed our world by combining keen observation of natural forces and practical methods to utilize that understanding. When our concept of electricity became more concise and comprehensive, we conceived and constructed an energy grid that distributes current, powering lights and appliances. We also built a vast telegraph network to send electrical signals over long distances, so we could communicate. Later, we invented telephones that used those same thin wires to encode our voices, enabling long distance conversations. Eventually, we invented computers and connected them to the extensive telephone circuits, giving rise to email and the internet. Science enables us to use our understanding of natural forces to build power

**Professor Zero:**

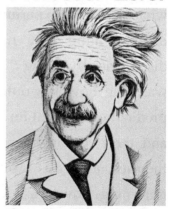

**Our Understanding Empowers Our Abilities**

grids and complex data networks. Our technologies evolve as our understanding grows, so as our awareness gets more precise, our skills improve. The strength of science is to quantify the external world of objective reality, using rulers and clocks. There aren't units to measure our internal experiences and abstract awareness. We can't quantify our consciousness. Without units, these concepts remain unscientific ideas, so we don't have formulas that capture the true nature of our internal, subjective world.

Fortunately for us, ancient traditions like Taoism and Ayurveda have highly refined concepts of our internal environments. They didn't build computers, but they developed sophisticated methodologies, like acupuncture, yoga, and meditation that explore our inner terrain and systematically harness human potential. We're able to blend the seemingly disparate perspectives of old and new into a unified vision of nature that includes the objective, outside world with the more subtle realms of personal experience. We keep the best of both: the rigor and discernment of science combined with an openness to explore inwardly. Sometimes, cutting edge research ventures beyond the concrete units of measurements that define our outer world.

Science and meditation both begin with impartial observation. We watch what happens. Experiments set up specific conditions that test our ideas, demonstrating how nature works. Einstein and Galileo made many discoveries by doing "Thought Experiments," envisioning a scenario and watching how it would play out. They blended intuition with logic to predict how natural forces operate, unleashing their imaginations to dream and then vetting their visions. Their open-mindedness saw beyond old theories and assumptions and revealed deep truths about nature, reframing how we view the world on a global level. These virtual experiments rewrote the laws of physics, and the new equations expanded our technology.

Healing is a personal *experiential experiment.* Your body and mind are the laboratory. This handbook is your lab manual, guiding your self-healing research with easy-to-follow meditations. When you absorb these concepts into your anatomy, you actualize your healing. Mental understanding isn't enough to change deep patterns; healing occurs when you *embody the understanding* and feel it in your bones. Reclaim your terrain and reinvent yourself from the inside out. When your inner experiences are grounded in reality, you gain traction and produce positive results.

The Quantum Needle Trilogy is a master class in self-healing. We begin with **Rebooting Your Nervous System**. Reducing tension helps you settle into yourself, sift through the noise, and find your safe place. Home base gives you the permission needed to detach deeply and dispel hyper-vigilance once and for all. Rebooting resets your adrenals and your vagus nerve, giving your BodyMind a chance to repair itself. Rebooting reframes past trauma, restoring harmony to the body, mind, and organs. It's a 2 step process:

> Step 1: **Unplug**
> Step 2: **Restart**

Step 1 of the Reboot is an electrical cleanse. Similar to a liver detox that clears molecular waste from your tissues, Rebooting your nervous system drains the excess electrical signals that clog your circuitry.

Step 2 occurs when you boot up a fresh circuit and restart a clean machine. Free from the residue of the past, your system implements your source code. Nature has programmed you to live, heal, fulfill your purpose, and manifest your best self. While this can seem daunting, rest assured that you're in good company because every living thing is striving to evolve After all is said and done, we all aspire to experience something interesting and express our unique selves.

Rebooting your nervous system clears your mind's neurological software. Chronic stress is a flaw in the circuitry where errant signals give your body's anatomical hardware the wrong instructions, causing inflammation. When inflammation becomes chronic, degenerative diseases degrade the body. Debugging your neural software restores the healthy programs that give your cells the right instructions. When your reactive fear response softens, you tap into your parasympathetic programming that cultivates health. Clearing the nervous system gives you a cohesive center and consolidates your Qi. The Reboot converts dysfunctional crashed loops into healthy *feedback* loops.

## Doctor Zero:

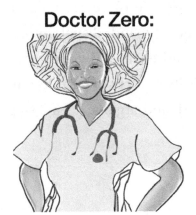

**Healing = Diagnosis + Treatment**

The Reboot Method develops your medicinal skillset. First, diagnose the problem. Second, provide medicine. Pain and symptoms show us where the body is blocked. Honest introspection and inner evaluation identify subtle wounds and crashed loops in the neural software. A detailed diagnosis also recognizes the causes of disease and maps out the mechanisms of the dysfunction. This understanding helps us find the right medicine for the condition we're facing. A deep Reboot gives you access to your blueprints so you can download the right code, restoring function to your many networks.

## Shaman Zero:

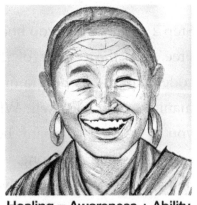

**Healing = Awareness + Ability**

Diagnosis and treatment can also be viewed as awareness and ability. Your *awareness* identifies where you're stuck, which activates your *ability* to implement the healing that's needed. Evolution teaches us to adapt by using our awareness to augment our abilities.

14

Integrating your sensory awareness gives you this actionable intelligence. Ideas aren't enough. Concepts become useful when they're digested, assimilated, and embodied. Awareness becomes ability when your experiences are somatically incorporated and internalized, when you embody the understanding. Your depth of feeling and capacity for SelfEmpathy gives your will its power.

Empathy is bonding and connecting to something or someone. When you empathize with a friend in trouble, you feel what they feel in your own body. By connecting directly, you know exactly how they hurt. Empathy diagnoses the problem by feeling into the wound and mapping it out. Your diagnosis is precise because you experienced the issue firsthand in your own tissue. The Reboot dares you to connect with every fiber of your body and every facet of your being, not just your intellect. When you empathically merge with your wounded parts, you *befriend* your trauma and reintegrate it. Befriending yourself cements the covenant of self, which compels you to help in any way. This impulse to help seeks the medicine that converts the malady into health. The diagnosis presents us with a challenge, and treatment is our response.

## Sensei Zero:

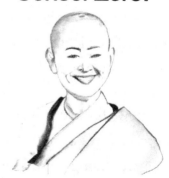

Healing = Empathy + Compassion

Compassion is the remedy that uses your empathic map of the wound to craft the cure. Once you connect from your heart, you'll do anything you can to serve the greater good. You'll give your dear friend your hard earned money or the shirt off your back. You'll gladly give a ride to the airport or be a devoted listener. Your complete devotion and commitment to your kin takes a "by any means necessary" strategy, and your empathy inspires compassionate actions. Rebooting builds your medicinal skills and refines your treatments.

Stem cells are master healers because they don't just throw medicine at the wound, they actually *become* the remedy. They embody medicine by transforming their body into the exact type of tissue that's been damaged. Stem cells are undifferentiated, so they are like a wild card in poker that can be any card that's needed. Once you bond and attain empathy, compassion arises naturally and you automatically become the wild card. Empathy diagnoses the cards in your hand, and compassion is how you become the joker, the ideal card. Rather than wait around and hope you are dealt a joker, you can train in the Reboot Method and build your stem cell skillset.

These advanced abilities are innate, but can be difficult to access, especially when your attention is consumed with the adrenal imperative of short-term survival, i.e. thinking and emoting. Getting stuck in the crashed loop of stress traps you in a vicious cycle. We don't escape or transcend these limiting patterns that lead to suffering; we go through them and restore functionality. When a vicious cycle spins in the other direction, it becomes a compassion cycle that continually feeds energy back in, amassing more energy and power. Feedback is how we rebuild our networks. To flip the script on the victim mindset, dive chest first into the unknown of your present moment, and let it flow right through you.

Every new discovery is a fresh way to see what nature has been doing all along. The laws of nature don't change or evolve, only our understanding gets clearer. Long before the wheel was invented, round rocks rolled down hills, and square rocks didn't roll as much. Inventing the wheel was just acknowledging the geometry of circles. Putting an axle in the center of the disk stabilizes the rotation, so you can make a cart or a bicycle. When your perspective grows, you see more of nature. As I treat patients and as I write this, I'm just uncovering what's right in front of us. As you read and implement the Reboot, you'll peel away layers of tension, revealing the real you that has always been there.

Defining the laws of physics on a macro level gives us a framework. As our understanding gets more precise on a micro level, our technology improves. The Reboot invites you to experience the laws of healing for yourself and incorporate these concepts into your corpus, your body. You can read about healing and memorize facts, but that won't empower you to upgrade your body's anatomical hardware and update your mind's neural software. Investigate for yourself, and live it. Direct experience uncovers your will, the motive force that propels change. Don't settle for mental reruns driven by a vague intent to heal; dare to shatter limitations and experience something new!

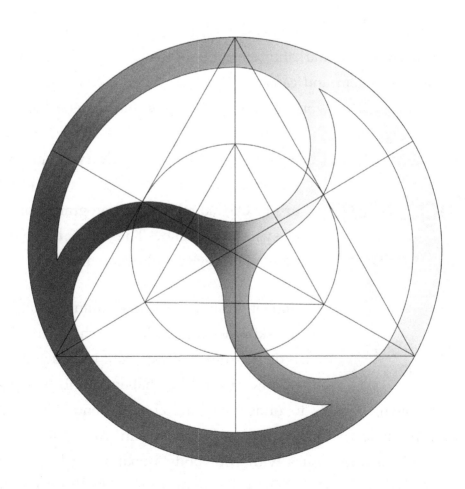

# Chapter Zero: Reboot Camp

When you turn on a computer, electricity starts flowing through the circuits and the machine activates its components. The processor fires up and deciphers data. Incoming signals enter the processor and outputs are sent to short-term memory or a hard drive that records everything. The keyboard gives you a way to interact and input your commands. The monitor reflects what's happening, so you can adapt your approach. Printers produce a document, a hard copy comprised of specific pixels. Each component plays a vital role and they all work together seamlessly.

If your computer crashes, you can turn it off and restart it. This simple reboot procedure is remarkably effective and clears most of the glitches that derail the system and cause it to freeze. When a computer engineer diagnoses a digital network, they find the bugs that impede the flow of data. If a program crashes, you can reboot it. When the whole system crashes, the problem is deeper than one program. Every program runs within the larger operating system (Windows or MacOS), so rebooting a program won't help a systemic crash. The first truth about networks: they're multilayered.

**Dig Deep!**

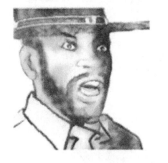

Reboot Camp is your basic training that instills the skills needed to identify where your flawed code is. Your Drill Sergeant impels you to step up and rise to the challenge. To debug your nervous system, it helps to understand the circuitry and the signals it conveys. You'll learn to pinpoint problems within your mind's neural software and identify issues with your body's anatomical hardware. To heal thyself, know thyself. The best way to understand the human nervous system is to fully occupy your own!

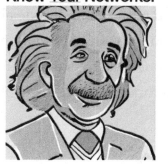

Your body is infused with about 65,000 miles (100,000 km) of nerves. These "wires" conduct current and convey signals to every part of you. Your nervous system is a complex data network that continuously communicates and talks with itself. Sensory nerves keep you informed: you perceive and become aware of your current circumstances. Motor nerves tell muscles to contract, enabling a response. Your neural circuit has electricity moving in two directions: toward the brain and away from the brain.

**Sensory = Inputs**. You have millions of sensors, allowing your skin to detect pressure, temperature, humidity, etc. Retinas detect visible light. Your nose has chemo-receptors that recognize certain aromatic chemicals in the air. When these sensors gets triggered, encoded messages are sent to your brain where they get processed and decoded. When your brain decodes electrical signals from your nose, you "smell" the molecules. There are so many incoming sensory signals that most of them get filtered and edited out before they get your attention. Your conscious awareness can only handle a small percentage of the immense volume of incoming information, so you're only getting a narrow bandwidth of what's happening. Rebooting filters out the noise and calibrates your sensory software so you get vital information.

**Motor = Outputs**. Motor nerves carry current from the brain to muscles, allowing you to move. When a motor nerve sends current to a muscle, the muscle contracts and gets shorter. This pulls on the bones and moves them. Muscles usually connect one bone to the next, so shortening muscles either bends or straightens the joint between the bones. Shortening the bicep bends the elbow while shortening your tricep straightens the arm.

**Feedback = Sensory + Motor.** The motor system enables you to respond to the information you got from your senses. After you receive and decode all the incoming signals, you can *do* something. You take in information, decode the data, and then you respond. The nervous system is an input-output machine: a network that gathers sensory information, processes it, and then arises at a motor response.

Combining incoming information and outgoing responses is powerful. The inputs pertain to awareness while responses are abilities. With each new moment, you get new and updated information, so you can adapt to different conditions. As you gather sensory awareness, your motor responses get smarter, and maybe even wiser.

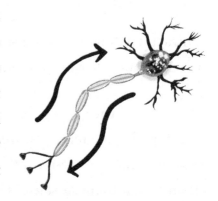

## Dimmer Switches

To better understand the motor system, imagine a dimmer switch and a light bulb. Adding current to the bulb makes it brighter. The dimmer lets you adjust exactly how much current you send, so you can fine tune the amount of light you want. Now picture a dimmer switch in your brain that controls a muscle. As you add current, you contract the muscle and shorten it. The more current you send, the shorter the muscle gets. If you turn the dimmer switch down, the muscle stops contracting and gets longer. Relaxed muscles are "off" and long. Muscles are like light bulbs because they both obey the signals they get. When given electricity, light bulbs change brightness while muscles change *length*.

You have hundreds of muscles in your body, and each one is controlled by a dimmer switch. There is a Dimmer Console in your brain with hundreds of dimmers. Every movement starts when you turn up a dimmer and send current to a muscle. When the muscle shortens, you move and you do something. It takes us years to learn how to use our dimmers and to develop motor control. Sometimes babies flail their arm and then seem surprised. They turned up a dimmer and triggered a contraction, but they didn't really know what would happen. It's as if the dimmer switches aren't labeled yet. It takes us years to stand on two legs and walk without falling. After years of training, we turn door knobs, feed ourselves, get dressed, brush our teeth, etc. Kids use the *hokey pokey* dance to test their dimmer skills: "Put your left foot in, put your left foot out, that's what it's all about." Motor control is a considerable task to manage, it's actually multi-tasking!

If you stand and lean a little, you have sensors that register you are tilting. You use this information to turn up the dimmers that align your skeleton vertically. Regaining your balance requires significant coordination between the incoming sensory data that tells you where you are in space, and the muscular responses that keep you upright. You need to shorten the right muscles at the right times to maintain your posture. Balance requires real-time updates and dynamic feedback.

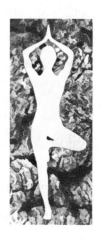

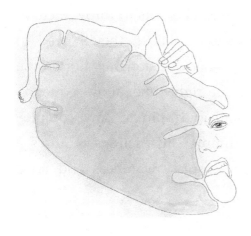

The Dimmer Console in your brain is called the homunculus. This weird cartoon shows an enlarged hand, face, and tongue, illustrating the fact that there are more dimmer switches to those areas. Your bicep is strong, but it's controlled by just one dimmer. Your hand has many small muscles, with many dimmers that add nuance to movement. The tongue also has many dimmers, so you can contract a region within the muscle. With many dimmers going to one muscle, you can control which fibers you shorten. Eating, talking, and swallowing require intricate contractions of portions of the tongue, and these fine-motor contractions need to be sequenced and timed. Deeper circuits including the vagus nerve and the autonomic system have a profound influence over our physiology and our state of being. When we Reboot these networks, we transform how our operating system operates.

## Technique = Dimmer Decisions

Let's say you want to play Chopin on the piano. To play each note you'll need to know how to move your fingers so you can hit the right key at the right time. You'll need to contract certain muscles in your forearm that pull on your finger bones, to push the piano 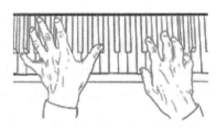 key. That means finding the specific dimmer switches that pull on those bones. You'll also want to use just the right amount of force so you can inflect the sound with artistry. It all boils down to **electrical choices**: where you send current, how much you send, and when.

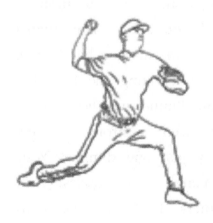 A pitcher in baseball wants to throw a curve ball. Similar to a pianist, they'll need to make good dimmer decisions to shorten the right fibers at the right time, all in sequence, to hurl the ball and spin it. Any complex sequence of dimmer instructions requires a high level of sensory awareness and crisp feedback.

Every movement is a dimmer decision. You make a multitude of electrical choices all the time. Are you aware of them? Most of us are too busy with other things to pay attention to our dimmer choices. If you're not occupied with the external world, you might be preoccupied with thinking. Chronic stress, muscle tension, inflammation, and pain reveal how the system has crashed. The Reboot is the remedy. The method is to actively attend to your Dimmer Console and reclaim command of your nervous system. Tension occurs when a dimmer is left on and the muscle continues contracting. The tight muscle is following orders and just doing what it's told to do. To effectively treat tension, we must address the source: too much current. We teach kids to turn off the light when they leave a room because it wastes power to have lights on for no reason. In your body, if you leave a motor dimmer on, you're wasting your energy with useless contractions.

**Choose your path to the Reboot Meditation**

If you want to skip ahead and listen to the Reboot Mediation audio now, go for it. Your Drill Sergeant gives you permission to bypass the rest of basic training temporarily, but after you experience the Reboot Meditation, resume reading from here. Otherwise, read on and finish Reboot Camp.

# Your New Normal is the Old You

Your engrained status quo that results from repeating the same thoughts, emotions, and behaviors is your new normal, even though it is not new at all. Once you get used to your persistent thoughts, your chronic emotions, and the habitual behaviors you repeat again and again, it is easy to space out and live by rote. Like a computer program running the same code over and over, habits are robotic. The Old You is a bunch of crashed programs that need an update. Rebooting is your reality check that refreshes your status quo and snaps you out of a rut.

All programs repeat, so repetition isn't the problem that makes us crash. Rituals are also repetitive behaviors, but participants try to sustain mindfulness by focusing conscious attention on the task at hand. In contrast, unconscious habits leak awareness. A deliberate Japanese Tea Ceremony builds presence, while impatiently waiting at a Starbucks drive-thru fragments you. The Reboot is a relaxation ritual. Beneath all the distractions, when your nervous system quiets down, your mind is actually clear. This crystalline clarity transforms the mundane into the NOW, and roots you in reality.

We are adaptable creatures, so we adapt to all kinds of circumstances. If you wear a watch every day, it'd feel strange to not have one on. *Habituation* is how we acclimate to things by doing them repeatedly, over and over. Smoking cigarettes is an example of fast habituation. When a person smokes a cigarette for the first time, their body initially rejects the smoke. They'll cough and gag because the lungs and membranes know the smoke is harsh and they don't want it. If a person persists and smokes again, they'll adapt and cough less. After about 10 cigarettes, they become a smoker, and their body acclimates to the smoke. The smoke is still toxic, and the cells do their best by adapting to the poison.

I've treated many smokers with acupuncture and the Reboot Meditation, and many reported that smoking made them physically sick after one treatment. Their body rejected the smoke, just like when they smoked that first cigarette. Long-time smokers suddenly realized their face smells like an ashtray! Rebooting reawakened the *inner non-smoker*, giving voice to that initial response that rejects toxic smoke, updating your sensory software.

Adapting is a double-edged sword. All species need to adapt to changing conditions, but habits can lull you into a dormant state. When you adapt and habituate to habits, you often lose conscious awareness. It's amazing how quickly people adapt to inhaling the smoke and soot of a burning cigarette. You have to become numb to the smell or you couldn't keep doing it. Becoming numb in this way is an example of a crashed loop that is out of touch with reality. The Reboot resets your sensory system, so you get the truth about what's happening. With accurate updates about the current reality, you can make a conscious choice.

There's no guarantee it'll be all roses. If there's a lit cigarette in your face, it's harsh. Once you awaken from the hypnosis that let you ignore the smell, you'll be motivated to get that fire and ash away from your face. It's remarkable how the non-smoker's body rejects the smoke by coughing and gagging while the smoker quietly smokes. Sometimes, having a dramatic reaction is better than staying silent, so symptoms aren't always bad.

Smoking helps illustrate these concepts, even though most of my patients have chronic inflammation, pain, and degenerative diseases. When symptoms become chronic, we have no choice but to habituate and adapt to being sick. Chronic pain quickly becomes deeply ingrained, and many of my patients are scared when they get better. It is so foreign for them to feel good; they're in disbelief, and they expect their old symptoms will return. People take comfort in what is familiar, even if it's crashed and unpleasant.

## EmoThinking

The Old You who's used to your not-so-new-normal has habituated to the way you view things and the way you feel about things. Your opinions and reactions seem automatic and built in, but they're also ingrained through repetition. The Old You doesn't notice the subliminal commentary coming from the voices in your head. It's so used to having the same thoughts and emotions, it doesn't even know it has any other options. Rebooting the Old You reveals how you've habituated to thinking the same thoughts and feeling the same way.

Most thoughts have an emotion linked to them, so most thoughts are really **EmoThoughts**. Our emotional energy merges with our mental energy, and unresolved emotions compel us to think the same things over and over. By and large, EmoThinking is a crashed loop driven by misguided survival instincts and overactive adrenals. In contrast, pure thinking is quite rare. Pure thought is contemplation, wondering how something works. Galileo and Einstein's thought experiments were inquisitive and open minded because they shed any emotional attachments to old beliefs, false assumptions, and obsolete ideas.

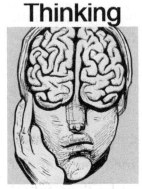

**Thinking**

**Stinks**

If we let go of our EmoThinking addiction even for a few moments, we give the "inner non-thinker" a chance to show itself. Just like the smoker who is no longer numb to how ashtrays smell, your inner non-thinker realizes the residue that EmoThinking creates is yucky. Especially when you think one thought after another, the "thought ashtray" overflows. The more you believe your thoughts, the more damaging they become. If you continue to feed energy into them, you double down on demise. EmoThinking can also throw your cells into a tailspin, increasing inflammation. To dismantle mental and physical stress, we need to get to the root cause.

## Stress = Excess Current

We all use the word stress, yet we rarely define it. In physics, when a force is applied to a material, it must adapt or it will break. The material experiences stress as it absorbs the force. Mechanical forces like weight compress a material, and if it can't hold the weight, it will buckle and break down. Other forces like electricity add charges to the material. Some stuff can handle extra electrons but other materials will heat up when saturated with current, burning up under the stress.

The stress we feel includes immune dysfunction and hormonal imbalance, but it's mostly an electrical overload. **Stress is too much current in the motor system**. The hallmark of stress is tension. These tight and shortened muscles are the result of too much current, caused by turning up dimmers and leaving them on.

Every time I assess a patient, I map out their tension pattern. This tells me which dimmer switches are too high (or too low), giving me the diagnosis of their dimmer console. Once I see where their system has crashed, I target my treatment and Reboot the crashed dimmers that are always on (or off).

Another consequence of this extra electricity is what I call **Neural Static**, background noise in the nervous system. Imagine how fluorescent lights buzz and flicker. When you charge a cell phone, the battery gets hot as the electricity moves. Large electrical transformers hum loudly as current passes through. After a rain, high-voltage electrical lines crackle. It's inevitable that there are side-effects as electricity moves, like noise, buzzing, flickering, or heat.

Neural static interferes with both mind and body. The noise and buzzing agitates the emotions and muddies neural software. Excess heat induces inflammation, like overheating a battery and damaging it. When cells follow the wrong code the physiology crashes, and the body's anatomical hardware suffers too. There's another consequence that's even more costly. White noise also interferes with sensory signals. How can we respond properly if the incoming data is incomplete, flawed, or corrupted by neural static?

# Neural Static

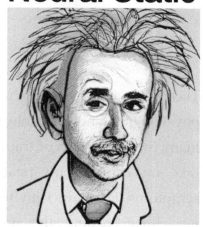

# Corrupts
# Sensory Data

The main commodity of the nervous system is electricity, which includes raw power and data. Sensory nerves inform us about what's happening inside and outside the body. Trying to have a conversation in a bustling restaurant is difficult if background noise blocks us from hearing. When we can't understand the incoming signals, we lose touch with what's happening. It's hard enough to hit a bull's eye, but it's even harder if we don't even know where the target is. Our sensory system gives us a reference point, so we can aim our attention and make our efforts effective.

Like our nervous system, cells also have feedback loops. When cells crash, they create chronic diseases, rampant inflammation, and psychological dysfunction. Cells make bad decisions when based on flawed information. You have more than a trillion cells that all work together. They're in constant communication with each other as they coordinate their activities to best serve you. Clearing neural static not only calms the mind, it also improves cellular synergy and efficiency.

Here's a short list of the consequences of stress:
- Tight muscles —> tension.  Orthopedic pain/joint compression
- Neural static —> mental stress.  Emotional/behavioral imbalance
- Inflammation —> cellular imbalance. Degenerative diseases
- Wasted resources —> depleting metabolic Qi.  Leaking LifeForce
- Corrupt sensory data —> we crash.  Freeze/out of touch

The wear and tear of chronic stress causes harm and amplifies the physiological and psychological symptoms that plague people. I've seen many manifestations of traumatic stress in my 30 years of clinical practice. Like any clinician, my treatments are judged by results i.e remission of symptoms. For now, I invite you to see beyond your symptoms, into the mechanism behind the problem. Especially with entrenched, chronic conditions, short-term relief and band-aids don't cut it. The more you hone in on the causes of dysfunction, the more you help yourself in the long run.

# Accuracy

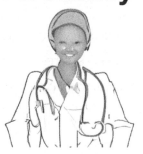

## Improves Outcomes

My acupuncture training included a metaphor about the root of a disease and the branches. Symptoms are the branches that we can see, and when we trace them down, they reveal the roots hidden below. Symptoms point us toward the flawed code that causes our condition and perpetuates our particular predicament, our pattern. If we are preoccupied with attacking symptoms rather than tracing them to the roots, we are stuck playing whack-a-mole. If we don't react to our circumstances, we can step back and get a global perspective. Once we identify the weak link, which might not be obvious at first, we can zoom in, get specific, and act locally. A comprehensive diagnosis reveals the root cause, and shows you your crashed code, the dysfunction driving the disease.

The Reboot Method guides you through your multilayered self, so you can get to the crux of your wounded parts. First, plug the leak and stop wasting energy on the crashed loops of stress. Rebooting also diverts your energy and attention back into you. This extra juice gets your systems up and running and restores feedback to your networks. The biggest insult to health is misusing our metabolic Qi energy. It takes energy to maintain chronic stress and inflammation, so not only does this damage the body and mind, it squanders precious Qi. It's a double whammy! Feedback feeds energy back into the system, converting chronic depletion into sustained nourishment. Reinvesting this energy inwardly empowers cells to make even more Qi. Channel this surplus, cellular energy back into your body to repair tissues and upgrade injured anatomical hardware. The Reboot Meditation recalibrates your neural software with functional programs that not only do their job, they even optimize cellular sustainability.

**Stress isn't neurological**

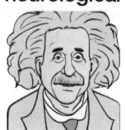

**It's neuro-illogical**

# Causes of Stress

Now that we have a definition of what stress is, and we surveyed the consequences of stress, let's tackle the question, "What drives stress and causes our nervous systems to crash"? The two main forces that create stress and turn up our dimmers are pain and adrenaline.

## Pain

When we feel a sensation we call pain, we turn up dimmers and tighten up. It's our natural defense, as if we're trying to block the pain, or support the wounded area. We immediately contract to try to guard or protect. Sending more current doesn't really help, it only makes our muscles tighter. If you have a pinched nerve that hurts and you add current to the muscles, the shorter muscles will crush down and further compress the nerve. This will undoubtedly hurt even more, which triggers you to turn up dimmers to cope with this stronger pain. This vicious cycle forges and escalates a chronic pain loop.

Tight muscles compress joints, which causes friction and contributes to arthritis. Perpetual tightness also blocks circulation, so the blood can't get through to carry away waste and bring oxygen and nutrients to cells. Muscles make lactic acid when they contract, so more contraction means more acid, which accumulates when the circulation is poor. Exercise also generates lactic acid, but the movement increases blood flow, which helps clear it. When you run, you contract and relax your muscles over and over, and your blood is pumping through. When you sit frozen at a computer, your muscles contract but don't lengthen. Over time, the fascial fibers lose elasticity and people get cemented into their overused position. If you experience pain and you are tempted to tighten up, please relax anyway. It's not fair, yet acceptance comes first. Resisting just adds current, even though the nerves are already saturated with too much current. Relaxing doesn't necessarily fix everything, but it doesn't make it worse. *Do no harm* is the first vow. Tightening just digs the hole deeper and adds to our burdens. For beginners, the Reboot Meditation can resolve mild to moderate pain. With practice, it can be helpful if things get worse, or go off the rails completely. Often, lengthening muscles does reduce nerve pain, quelling the fire. Numerous patients and students have commented that they had reduced pain after a Reboot, and many attained long-term remission.

**Adrenaline**

Adrenaline is the other driver that cranks up our dimmers. The fight-or-flight response is our reaction to feeling threatened. To get safe you'll run or fight your way out of danger. *Freeze* is another important adrenal response, so it's really freeze, flight, or fight. The freeze response is a state of shock, like the deer in the headlights syndrome. Freeze can be helpful to a rabbit hiding from a predator, remaining quiet and still but also braced and ready to run full speed at any second. Like a sprinter waiting for the starting gun or a boxer waiting for the bell, the entire system is fully charged and ready to react at any moment.

All 3 adrenal options activate your motor side. To run as fast as you can, you'll need all the electricity you can get, immediately. Fighting requires stronger contractions to forcefully move your bones to defeat your opponent. You need all the current you can get and you need it NOW. **Adrenaline turns up every dimmer and causes every muscle to contract.** With fight or flight, the adrenaline is channeled into moving the body, either running or fighting your way to safety. The energy gets used. If you survive the ordeal, the fight-or-flight reaction paid off, and you can relax again because the threat has passed. The freeze response doesn't discharge the extra current through the physical body. The energy gets retained and diverted toward the mind: it propels thinking and ruminating. **Excess**

**mental energy and EmoThinking are driven by the trapped energy of the freeze response**. Adrenaline spins a web of noise in your head, keeping you occupied so you are, in effect, frozen. Most of us are preoccupied most of the time, so we're in a semi-frozen and dissociative state! When you think the same thoughts over and over, you're chasing your tail and caught in a crashed loop.

Just like the chronic pain loop, adrenaline and thinking feed each other and create a vicious cycle. Thinking perpetuates the fear response which includes secreting more adrenaline. Getting whipped up in a mental frenzy stimulates the body to secrete even more adrenaline. This extra adrenaline accelerates thoughts and inflames emotions. People become even more anxious, setting the stage for a panic attack.

The **Pain Loop:** The more pain you feel, the more you turn up your dimmers, which causes more pain, so you turn up dimmers even more.

The **Adrenal Loop:** The more you think, the more adrenaline you secrete, causing you to think faster, triggering the adrenals, speeding up thoughts.

These are the two big pitfalls that derail neural software and block your electrical Qi circuit. If you experience pain or adrenaline for a week or two, you adapt to that toxic condition, like becoming a smoker. You turn up dimmers and get used to your not-so-new normal. Crashed loops become chronic and familiar. If you're in pain, ill, or worried, if you have a deadline or if your friend is having a crisis, you're continually amping up your dimmers. Pretty soon they're all higher than they need to be. More pain or adrenaline will turn up the dimmers a bit more, until that becomes the next new-normal. After a while, your baseline dimmers are too high and your motor is revving constantly. After you adapt to adrenal stress, you forget you can reduce your idle speed.

Let's look at 3 ways you can lengthen a muscle:

-Massage

-Stretch

-Turn off the Dimmer …. aka Relax

Massage and acupressure involve *pressing* on the tissue, which often helps muscles relax. Stretching is *pulling* on the muscle and forcing it to lengthen. Both pressing on muscles and pulling them apart focuses the attention on the muscle. Turning off the dimmer focusses on the switch that commands the muscle. Muscles are like light bulbs and they don't decide what they do. They don't get to pick if they're on or off. What they do depends entirely on the current they receive.

Your muscles are dutifully obeying the dimmers that control them. They contract only when commanded by the motor signal. That's good news, because you can turn off any dimmer switch that tells its muscle to contract. Why is the muscle contracting and tight in the first place? It's always the same answer: the switch is on.

There can be a million reasons *why* you left the dimmer on, but regardless of the reason, you can now focus your complete attention on turning that switch off. Any time you feel tension and you want to stretch or massage a muscle, remember that it's tight because you're telling it to tighten. You can press it and pull it all day, but until you turn off the dimmer switch in your brain, the muscle won't really let go. As soon as you stop sending electricity, the fibers release and lengthen immediately, barring dehydration and electrolyte imbalance. If massaging tight muscles helps you turn off the dimmer, great. Hopefully your system learns how to keep that dimmer off. Here's the rub: if your new normal includes your dimmers being on, then the muscle will have no choice but to tighten up again when you unconsciously turn up dimmers. Rebooting doesn't focus on muscles, we go straight to the source: the switches.

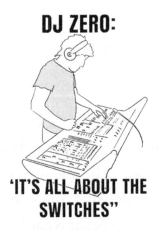

**DJ ZERO:**

**'IT'S ALL ABOUT THE SWITCHES"**

When you turn a light off, you don't usually unscrew the light bulb or throw a towel over the lamp to block the light. You turn off the switch instead. Every move you make demonstrates your control over your dimmers; you turn the current up or down to meet the needs of any given moment, all day long. You call the shots! Reclaim control of your very own electrical grid by Rebooting the switchboard, the Dimmer Console in your brain. It might seem contradictory, but I hope you're excited to relax!

## The Adrenal Spectrum

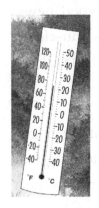

Picture the adrenal spectrum as a vertical thermometer. Rather than measuring thermal energy as degrees of temperature, this device measures adrenaline and your level of safety. Your adrenals are programmed to ascertain if you are safe or threatened so they constantly ask, Friend or Foe? Just like Celsius and Fahrenheit accurately measure hot and cold, your adrenal spectrum defines exactly how safe you are.

Your safety includes your physical safety in your environment and how safe you *feel*. At any time you can assess your level of real world, objective safety and your degree of internal, subjective safety. The top part of the spectrum has the heightened adrenal states, all the way to extreme panic and shock. As we go lower, there's less adrenaline, and we're more relaxed. At the bottom of the spectrum, the entire motor system is off. Soon you'll unplug your muscular motor machine for a full reboot.

We move up and down the spectrum throughout the day. When someone is threatened or has a sharp pain, they secrete adrenaline and jump into action. Fight or flight only works when you respond quickly, so adrenaline ensures we turn up dimmers and escalate contractions immediately. When a person feels relief, they relax and move down on the spectrum. It often takes a bit longer for your biochemistry to descend, but I'll show you the short cuts! After their first successful Reboot, people are surprised by how quickly they descended down the spectrum and are amazed by how deeply they let go.

## The trick is to feel, not think...

When you feel, you take your temperature and locate where you are on the spectrum. As you settle into your sensory side, you get your bearings and find your center. Now your senses can make sense of things. Feeling takes your mindfulness to the next level because you get a full body, somatic experience. You're not just paying attention; you're actively processing your sensory signals. This grounds you in reality and connects you to your Here and your Now.

When your location gets locked in, you realize there's no reason you have to be at this exact spot on the spectrum. You have some control and some command over your reality, so you can sink down a bit. While our circumstances influence us profoundly, we also have a modicum of free will. When you're in a pain loop or an adrenal loop, you're spinning your wheels. Crashing makes you forget you have choice, so you get stuck in repetitive EmoThought loops. **Your sensory skills help you find your will and access its power.** How? Knowing where you are plants you on solid ground and gives you a foothold. You gain traction, so you can move forward. Rather than flailing around aimlessly, your efforts become effective, and you exert a force in the real world.

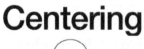

# Centering

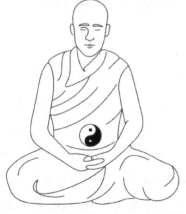

## Consolidates Will

The Reboot invites you to take stock and reclaim your dimmers. You have the power to move down a notch. You might even sink down ten levels. You could be more relaxed than you've ever been, and then drop down even more. There's always a level beneath you! Feeling is the key that opens you and EmoThinking is the lock that restrains you. Thinking moves you up on the spectrum and activates the motor system. EmoThinking is actually a frozen state, which turns up dimmers to prepare you for flight or fight. While consumed in this fictitious daydream, your muscles get tighter and your body suffers. Even though you are not physically moving, your body is all amped up. This overheats the brain and disorganizes the organs, inflaming mind and body. Thinking makes you red line and Rebooting cools your jets. Take this offramp and chillax!

## Reboot Your Motor Side

Unplugging a computer empties the circuits and clears the residue of all the data that has been processed. A Reboot doesn't mean you forget because your data is saved; it's more like you come to terms with what happened, and you actually process it. This frees up your processor, defragments your hard drive, and recalibrates your operating system. The Reboot drains the energy that propels the crashed loops we call stress. Technically speaking, rebooting the nervous system means unplugging the motor side. We keep the sensory side open to feel what's happening, and we use that insight to let go even more.

The sensory side shuts off when we're unconscious, either asleep or anesthetized. While awake, we can't really turn off the sensory side: we hear what we hear, and we feel what we feel. We can interpret these signals in different ways, but the data goes to the brain and gets processed. If we could block sensory signals, we wouldn't need pain medication because we would just block the signal before it got to the brain to be interpreted as pain. We typically don't have that luxury when we're awake. Rebooting the motor side means turning every dimmer to zero, unplugging the muscles, and relaxing the body. Take a fresh look at your dimmers to be sure they're off, and not just at their "new normal" version of off. Just as a smoker can tolerate tar and soot in their sinuses, you can acclimate to tight muscles and ignore the neural static that disturbs your nervous system. Both are repugnant, but you only realize it when you step outside of the unconscious pattern and regain your perspective.

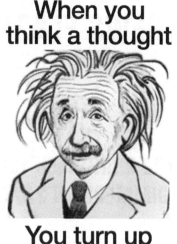

**When you think a thought**

**You turn up a dimmer**

How does the "Inner Non-Thinker" awaken? Clearing neural static makes you aware that EmoThinking has a similar tar-like residue that gums up your mind's neural software. It's time to enlist and sign your name on the dotted line by committing to turning off your muscles completely. Rather than turning off the sensory side by numbing out or checking out, we're going to check in. We actively open to the incoming data stream and feel all of it. Now you'll know for sure if the dimmers are truly off. You can't just assume they're off; you need to **feel and verify.**

## Relaxing = AntiTechnique = NonDoing

Feel, don't do. The first skill is to separate the sensory side from the motor side. The Reboot Method is to turn off your motor side and actively open the sensory side. Are you focused on perceiving incoming sensory information, or are you responding with your motor side by turning up dimmers? Holding this awareness is fundamental. Rather than responding and trying to fix your flaws, your new goal is to **notice and witness where your attention is**. This helps you recognize when you react, so you can bring your attention back to the sensory side.

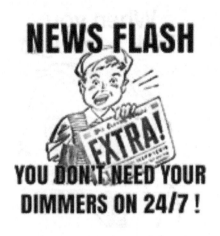

**NEWS FLASH**

**YOU DON'T NEED YOUR DIMMERS ON 24/7 !**

All technique gets suspended and we are no longer interested in doing anything. Everything you *do* starts as a dimmer signal that shortens a muscle and pulls on a bone, causing a physical action. Relaxing shuts off the motor side, so we can apply all of our attention to the sensory side. This allows you to feel whether the dimmers are off or not. With no tasks to complete, you don't need to breathe deeper, move your skeleton, play the piano, throw a curve ball, or even blink. If you endeavor to turn off every dimmer, you're committing to not doing anything.

## Muscles are *Anti-Gravity Devices*

Gravity is always there, pulling everything straight down. In order to lift your heavy bones, you need to exert a force that's stronger than gravity. Movements begin by turning up dimmers, shortening muscles, pulling on bones, and bending joints. Moving requires muscles that are strong enough to overpower gravity.

When there's no electricity going to a muscle, it lengthens and stops pulling on the bones. Fun fact: **relaxing is letting go of your bones**. Relaxing is giving your bones to gravity and allowing it to simply pull the body downward. Muscles are anti-gravity devices that lift heavy bones against the gravitational pull. When you shut off a dimmer switch, you allow gravity to have that bone and pull it straight down. If you shut off all the dimmers for your whole body, you let go of your entire skeleton! Chapter 3 includes a series of Trust Fall Meditations that build the permission needed to fully surrender to gravity and release physical tension.

# Building Trust Is Getting To Yes

Are you living with an overactive mind, shortened muscles, and lots of neural static? If relaxing were easy, I'd write a different book. **Relaxing requires you to summon your will and assert command of the dimmer console in your brain.** The dimmers and muscles are yours, but stress distracts you, so you lose control. If you let your EmoThinking mind whisper in your brain all day and night, telling you to turn up dimmers because you might be threatened somehow, you are in an Adrenal Crashed Loop. Freeze, Flight, and Fight are loops that generate momentum, so they tend to keep going. They won't stop by themselves, and they won't stop because you don't like the consequences. Inertia only changes when acted upon by an outside force. You are the only one who can stop the vicious cycle of chronic stress. How? Withdraw the electricity that fuels it. It's time! Choose to unplug from it for a while. See what happens. If your habits aren't producing good results, back off and take a fresh look. There's no guarantee you will get a breakthrough, but your odds improve exponentially when you tap your will to let go and Reboot!

## You Are Under No Contract

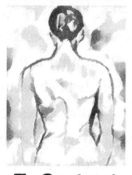

## To Contract Your Muscles

At this moment, you don't need to commit to unplugging forever. You just need to let go for a short time. Just let go NOW. Don't worry about the future. You don't need to buy into some religion, believe in metabolic Qi energy, or adopt some spiritual paradigm. When I treat a smoker who wants to quit, I ask them why. If it's because their spouse coerced them, or they "should" for their health, I immediately inform them that this motivation simply won't cut it. My favorite answer is when a patient says something like, "I'm over it," or "I'm really sick and tired of it." They've done it enough and they wore it out, so there is nothing redeeming left. They are no longer debating, overthinking, or overly emotional about it. They are at rock bottom. Most of my patients have seen many other doctors and therapists before they come to me, so they are desperately seeking relief and willing to venture into the unknown.

If you are wishy-washy, the inertia of the dysfunctional crashed loops overrides the *attempt* to change. Intentions and trying are useless if they are not backed up with your will. You deepest motivation has the power to exert enough force to alter the inertia of your chronic pattern. Most people think of rock bottom as a bad place, but I see it as the turning point, the point of inflection, when you change direction. Rather than self-destruct, you feed constructive energy back into yourself. Healing occurs when a crashed loop is converted into a feedback loop, when a vicious cycle becomes a compassion cycle. In this context, rock bottom is when healing begins.

Stress is an adrenal addiction. Thinking too much, especially thinking the same thoughts over and over, means you are not just a casual user. Your emotions provide your biochemical fix, and you secrete the dopamine and hormones that you depend on to feel normal. There are many imbalances of overuse: being a workaholic, rageaholic, alcoholic etc. Underachievers are also tied to the tragic tale of being a loser, a persona that haunts many people. Bad things happen that hurt good people, but buying into being a victim of circumstances is one of the most pervasive and limiting beliefs that fuels stress. Once you adopt the storyline and you believe your EmoThoughts, you drink the Kool Aid and allow your circumstances to define who and what you are. Believing your EmoThoughts often disempowers you and feeds energy into the debilitating vicious cycle we call the Ego. Rock bottom is the moment you stop repeating your Ego's crashed loops. You unplug and complete Step 1 of the Reboot. Step 2 restarts your fresh circuitry, and you take your first willful step toward YES.

# Sensory Skills

Consider the hours that athletes, musicians, soldiers, and dancers spend training their motor skills, perfecting their exceptional technique. With full command of their dimmers, they move in precise ways at will. With rigorous training and expert coaching, they also develop incredible stamina. Runners build strong legs and lungs, upgrading their anatomical hardware. Imagine that same investment of time and attention given to training the sensory side. What skills could you develop if you trained your senses?

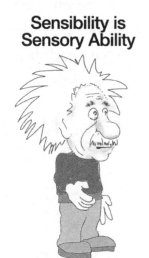

**Sensibility is Sensory Ability**

**It's Common Sense**

As we keenly listen to the body, and feel into our condition, we get better information about what's happening. We develop our awareness of our self and our surroundings, dialing in to what is going on inside us and around us. We get our bearings, which helps us adapt appropriately. If our senses are cloudy or muddled with neural static, we lose touch and we also lose function.

Your somatic sensory skills are the foundation of your motor talents. Science teaches us that awareness augments ability! The more deeply we understand natural forces, the more we can channel nature's energy. Your sensibility, your ability to sense what is happening, helps you perform optimally. When your senses provide accurate information, your motor system sends better dimmer signals. Cells also excel when they get the best instructions. Otherwise, they veer off track and crash, causing inflammation.

Reboot Camp trains your sensory skillset by asking you to assess where you are on the Adrenal Spectrum. At any time, your Drill Sergeant can demand a *Dimmer Status Report*. This isn't a conversation about why you are stressed out, it is a concise report of your motor status. Period. Your explanation and narrative about your dimmer choices are not relevant now, and we will address that later. Now that you are enlisted as a Reboot foot soldier, you must march mindfully and surpass your previous limits.

**Sensory Stamina**

When you sink into your sensory side, and you decline EmoThinking, you don't just map out your dimmers, you stop feeding the pain loops and adrenal loops that turn them up. If you stay with feeling and you don't get sucked back into your head, you sustain your sensory attention. Each moment you decline reacting reinforces your sensory stamina, so you maintain mindfulness for the extra mile. Each step onward, and each little success, consolidates your commitment and ability to follow through.

You can't graduate from Reboot Camp until you make it through the infamous obstacle course. Picture a military obstacle course that confronts you with crawling through mud, climbing ropes, scaling walls, running, getting yelled at, carrying heavy weight, etc. When your life confronts you with a barrier, are you going to throw in the towel and whine about how 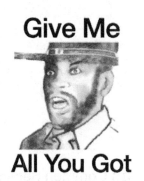 **Give Me**

**All You Got**

high the wall is or how dirty the mud is? Welcome to the world of "no excuses!" You either meet the moment you are in or you get derailed. You either process what is happening or you EmoThink about it. Healing hinges upon the ability to surmount the illness, and medicines are judged by whether they work or not.

I didn't make the rules about the survival of the fittest, which is life's obstacle course. Nature gives each of us talents and flaws, and it is our choice to either devote ourself to developing our skillset or make excuses and pay lip service. The binary question is: are you an active participant or a spectator? This is the line between intention and will, distinguishing wishful thinking from actually giving your all to advance beyond the barrier. Intention is an attempt and will pulls all the stops to make it happen.

Most cadets slip when they first try scaling the wall. Sincerely wanting to succeed doesn't magically give them the necessary skills. Maybe they can't grip the rope tightly enough or dig their toe into a crack to get a firm footing. Without a foundation, they can't climb. After slipping around and getting frustrated, a good cadet works to solve problems and find a way. If they recognize the importance of building grip strength and learning how to use the tip of their boot to find something stable to climb on, they will make progress. To succeed, they need the where-with-all to focus on their connection to the rope to "get a grip" and find their footing to "get grounded." Getting centered gets them on the right track.

Your persistent and consistent focus makes you stronger so you can handle the hurdles. It takes tenacity to build skills. As soon as you revert to EmoThinking, neural static become yet another obstacle that blocks you from focussing on your foothold. Holding your attention on the sensory side clears the neural static that interferes with your perception. With less brain fog, you can identify your "flaws" and see exactly what you need to do to restore function and manifest your vision.

You can't traverse life's obstacle course if you are afraid of failure. Shame motivates certain behaviors but doesn't inspire creativity or healing. Your true motivation isn't about proving you are good enough, it's about finding your place in the world and tapping the Qi energy that animates you and brought you this far. When you experience physical or emotional pain, it's even more important that you release tension and break the pain loop. Deep relaxation goes beyond hovering on the surface. The more current you withdraw, the more beneficial your Reboot is. When you genuinely let go and surrender, your system quiets down and your senses aren't clouded by all the noise. This awakens intuition and fosters "a-ha" moments. You learn more about yourself, and these insights amplify your effectiveness.

## Permission

Adrenaline is there to keep you alive, so it makes a compelling case. Relax? If your life is at stake, you'd better jump! Relaxing would be ignoring the warning that your cells feel when there's lots of adrenaline around. Adrenaline alerts you of danger so you can respond quickly and get back to safety. It's a great failsafe to help keep you alive, but it's overdeveloped and misused. Believing in false threats gets you all worked up. When distracted, you ignore the actual problems you face, making you ill-equipped to deal with the reality you're in.

To let go, you have to **overtly receive permission to override the adrenal warning**. If you're clenching your teeth, or stressing in any way, your dimmers are too high and your electrical Qi is imbalanced. When you receive permission to relax, you are released from any obligations to remain vigilant, allowing you to soften. Until you get permission, you are still on the hook and not yet willing to fully surrender. Your safety isn't real yet. It's a nice idea, but platitudes are hollow words that ring empty. The moment you feel safe, you embody the understanding of what it means to be safe. You experience safety for yourself, directly in your own body, right HereNow! When theory becomes reality, your intelligence becomes actionable.

If you are frozen with adrenal fear, don't *try* to relax. If you don't have permission yet, accept the fact that you are not ready to let go. Stop trying and concede that this isn't your breakthrough moment. It's ok to fall short. This is not the first time a living person was imperfect, and it is not last time. Forgive yourself for failing to measure up. Sometimes, realizing that trying is a dead end actually opens the door. When there's an opening, give yourself permission to go a little farther, and release something. Permission allows you to step beyond adrenal concerns, expanding your exploration of the vast and remarkable world within you. When you notice you're trying, grant yourself permission to just be with your angst.

Instead of trying to find your zen, commit to opening your sensory side and feeling the moment you are in. Dare to challenge the impulse to tighten and constrict. Give yourself permission to feel your tension and relax. With steady resolve, resist being enticed to turn up a dimmer for no *real* reason. Once you see that each EmoThought is an excuse keeping you sucked into drama, you gain the authority 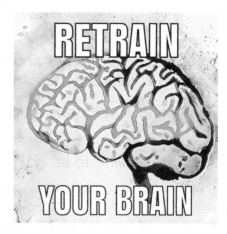 to override it. You outrank that voice in your head so you can decline to indulge your emotional impulses. If you want more control over your health and circumstances, get control of your dimmers. Don't let your EmoThinking Ego dictate your dimmer decisions!

If you're fretting about what already happened or worried about what might happen, you're ignoring the present moment. Another byproduct of this delusion is turning up dimmers. Tightening a muscle doesn't help you solve mental stress. We're drawing a line in the sand and turning our dimmers off NOW! There's no good reason why you can't do that, even if your mind tells you that you shouldn't let go. Claim this moment to show up and shut down. Permission empowers your will to let go. Letting go sounds passive, but you actively overriding your EmoThinking survival programming. Trust gives you the clout to not take the bait. Voluntary movement is different from reflexes because you make a conscious choice. The word "volition" pertains to the will, the part of you that makes things happen. Every time you turn up a dimmer on purpose, your will commands it and the electricity is sent. It works the other way too: every time you turn a dimmer OFF on purpose, your will commands it. Letting go is an act of will, a conscious choice.

## You Have the Right to Relax

- Turning up a dimmer and lifting your arm is a voluntary action.

- Relaxing is voluntary *inaction*, an act of will.

- Are you *willing* to let go?

- You have the right to remain silent…

- Anything you let go of cannot be used against you…

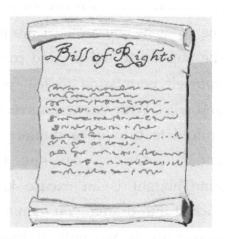

Your Reboot Camp Drill Sergeant challenges you to relax more than you ever have. Whatever degree of release you consider to be your deepest experience of surrender, there is always a level below that you could sink into. How far are you willing to go? How committed are you? How much healing are you ready for? Can you handle the truth? It's up to you.

Deep detachment fosters dreams and conveys insights. Letting go in this way allows your perspective to grow. Once you regain control of your Dimmer Console, you realize that you command your muscles. Suddenly, you have more options. A crashed computer is stuck in a rut, repeating the same limited code. Thinking the same things over and over gives you tunnel vision, distracting you from your own will, your personal power. Any trauma, physical injury, or psychological abuse becomes neural static and clogs your circuits. Feedback breaks down and you crash, physically or mentally. The Reboot clears your nervous system and centers you.

# THE REBOOT MEDITATION

Now it's best to switch to audio and listen to the guided Reboot Meditation. Use www.RebootYourNervousSystem.com or the QR code on the inside cover. Recline or lie down face up with your legs elevated. The most important skill is to NOTICE whether your attention is on your sensory side or your motor side. Are you FEELING, or are you DOING? Lie down or recline, settle in, and get as comfortable as possible. Listen.

Notice your body and any sensations you're feeling. Draw your attention to the parts of your body that move as you breathe. Just witness and watch your body while it's breathing. As you tune in to your breathing, notice if you're tempted to *do* something to your breath. Often, we judge our breath as shallow, and so we try to correct the shallowness by taking a deep breath. We immediately go from the sensory side to the motor side. We stop observing the breath, and we jump right into a correction. Every dimmer signal you send is an instruction, telling a muscle to shorten and perform an action. Our goal with the Reboot is to turn the entire motor system off.

Notice how the breath moves through your body. Perhaps your abdomen rises and falls, maybe your ribcage moves as well. Wherever you feel that movement, imagine a balloon located there. Just like a regular balloon, your "breathing balloon" is made of a thin elastic material that stretches as it inflates. When a balloon deflates, it implodes and retracts toward the hollow center. Anatomically, we have two lungs in the ribcage. When the diaphragm pulls downward, air is drawn into the chest. Picture a single balloon slightly lower than your actual lungs, that fills with air and empties. When you inhale, your balloon inflates and expands. The elastic membrane pushes outward in all directions equally, and the ball gets bigger, expanding in all 3 dimensions.

Picture the top and bottom of the balloon. As the balloon inflates, feel the top of the balloon move up toward your collarbones, while the bottom of this elastic skin drops down toward the pelvis. During inhalation, the balloon gets taller vertically. As the body exhales, the balloon shrinks. The top and bottom retract toward each other, toward the center of the balloon.

Now, consider the front and the back of your breathing balloon. As the balloon fills, the front of the balloon pushes toward the ceiling, lifting the belly and chest outward. At the same time, the back of the balloon is pressing toward the floor. When you inhale, the back half of the balloon is expanding toward the spine and toward the kidneys. This region, the back of the balloon, is a very important part of your body. As the balloon inflates, feel the back of the balloon as it expands toward the kidneys. Allow your attention to stay connected to this place, the back half of the balloon. As the balloon changes size, watch how the thin, elastic skin of the balloon interacts with the front of the spine.

Even though you're focussed on this location, you don't need to *do* anything. No muscles are necessary. You can just observe and witness the breath come and go. At any time, refocus and bring your full attention to the back part to the balloon. If you're tempted to *do* something, you're trying to change something. Instead of implementing your idea of a correction, turn off your dimmers and let go. Point your attention at that exact thing you want to change and accept it. Rather than react with your motor system, use your sensory side to just feel it. Accept this moment you're in and experience the sensations you are receiving. Commit to listening, regardless of the circumstances.

Watch the balloon as it fills and empties. If you notice tension, turn off the dimmers that are telling those muscles to contract. Rather than doing something to compensate for tension, feel what's happening there. Turn off the dimmer switches and relax that area. Especially notice how the back of the balloon inflates and presses toward the front of the spine, toward the kidneys.

Now picture a hollow tube that extends upwards from the balloon. It passes up through the chest and continues through the throat. It winds through the skull, opening at the nose and mouth. This tube is the airway. Incoming air fills your balloon. When your balloon retracts, air moves up the tube and out of the body. If you're breathing through your nose, you can follow your inhale up the nose to the area between you eyes. The air then moves back and down, passing through the sinuses behind your face, through the throat, and all the way down to the inflating balloon. As the balloon deflates it pushes the air back up the tube, from the body to the head, and then out through the nose or mouth.

The throat region is a series of valves. We can divert air through the nose or the mouth, altering the passageway. We can divert our exhale through the vocal cords to rattle them and make sound. We can also by-pass the voice box and just exhale quietly. There's also a flap for the esophagus, another tube which is for eating and drinking. With all of these flaps and valves, the air going in and out of the balloon has to go through an obstacle course to get through the throat. Any tension here makes the tube a little more narrow, which limits air flow. Relaxing your tongue and opening your throat allows the balloon to move air more easily. Open the airway and feel the balloon fill and empty with less resistance.

The tongue as a muscle like any other, with a dimmer in the brain that controls it. We're mostly interested in the back of the tongue, where the tongue becomes the throat. We're less concerned with the tip of the tongue. As you start to find the dimmers that control the throat and the underside of your chin, you might notice your jaw relax. As the tongue releases, the jaw tends to drop, and the mouth might hang open. Give yourself permission to allow the chin to fall. As the muscles get longer, you can feel the tube in the throat get larger, increasing in diameter. As the tube opens, air moves more easily.

With the open throat, watch the balloon as it fills and empties. You might notice changes. Just by releasing the throat and opening the tube, the breath might slow down. It might get quieter or softer. It might get deeper. Whatever you notice continue to feel the back of the balloon. If you're tempted to do something, listen more precisely and feel what's happening there. Whatever you want to change, accept it instead. Rather than try to change it, allow it to be what it is and relax anyway.

NOW, bring your attention to the dimmers in your brain. You operate a large console with hundreds of dimmers, one for every muscle. Any time you turn up a dimmer switch, you send current to that muscle and you shorten it. This pulls on the bones and moves the body. Every action you've ever done began when you sent electricity to a muscle.

Your dimmer console in your brain includes a master switch. Like a circuit breaker or a power switch, this dimmer controls the entire panel. This master switch controls all the dimmers, so it controls every muscle in the body. As you're ready, NOW, turn off this master switch. Shut off the electricity to all the muscles and allow them to lengthen. Soften and relax.

As your muscles release and lengthen, they stop pulling on the bones as if to move them. This gives them to gravity, which takes the weight and draws it downward. You might actually feel this as heaviness or as a sinking sensation. It's simply gravity acting on your tissues and pulling them down. You are safe now. Sink into the support beneath you and let it hold you.

You might also notice that the balloon continues to fill and empty, on its own, illustrating that the body maintains itself. You don't have to *do* anything. You can relax even more, sink even deeper, and allow even more current to be diverted away from the muscles. **Chime ends the meditation.**

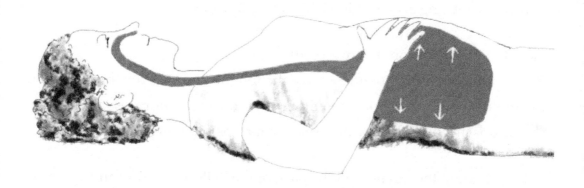

Rest quietly for as long as you like. It's OK to fell asleep. When you're ready, refocus your attention and feel how your balloon and tube move air. Especially notice any tension in the tongue and feel the back of the balloon as it inflates toward your spine and kidneys. If your mind conjures up thoughts and emotions, you don't need to respond to them right away. Keep your attention on the tube and the balloon, especially the throat and the back of the balloon.

To re-emerge into a normal waking state, you don't have to do much. Slowly move your fingers and toes and notice how the balloon keeps operating on its own. Notice your tongue and check to see if it's still relaxed. As soon as you think a thought, you turn up a dimmer. Often the tongue is among the first muscles you constrict when EmoThoughts distract you or when pain inflames your nervous system.

# Reboot Refresher

Notice the breath: don't respond, react, or intervene. Just notice. Stay with your sensory side and feel what's happening. To Reboot the motor side, turn off your dimmer switches and stop doing. See and feel the Balloon and Tube, noticing all sensations, including tension.

**Task 1:** Relax your tongue to open the tube.
Release the root of the tongue, where the tongue becomes the throat. Soften the underside of chin. You can still breathe through your nose even if the chin drops. It's ok if the jaw drops and your lips separate a little.

**Task 2:** During the inhale, feel the back of the balloon as it expands.
Feel and see the back part of your elastic balloon expanding toward the floor. The back of the balloon massages the kidneys and the front of the lower spine.

**Helpful Hint:**
Putting one hand on your abdomen and the other on your chest helps you map out the front of your balloon as it inflates. Because your balloon is 3D, when the front pushes toward the ceiling, the back of the balloon pushes toward the spine. Use your hands as sensors that detect the subtle movements as the breath moves through your torso.

**Task 3:** Turn all dimmers off.
Give yourself permission to let go. Shut off one dimmer at a time. As you notice tension, relax it. Use the *master dimmer switch* in the brain to shut off all the muscles. If you are EmoThinking, bring your attention back to your sensory side. The more you feel, the more you relax.

# Medical Debrief: Health Benefits of the Reboot

    1) More Oxygen
    2) Dismantle Stress
    3) Spinal Breathing

1)    Oxygen might be important…perhaps. Our concept of nutrition centers around eating food to give our cells the molecules they need to thrive, yet I recognize that $O_2$ is the primary nutrient cells need. Your cells need protein, fats, and carbs, but their most immediate requirement is oxygen. The mitochondria within cells produces our metabolic energy (ATP) in a process called *cellular respiration.* It's interesting that biochemists call this respiration because it implies that cells are breathing. The word Qi translates as *energy and breath,* an ancient way to describe this same process of cellular respiration. Just like a fire needs ventilation, your metabolic engine needs air flow. Improve your diet by breathing freely!

2)    How do we dismantle stress?
    -The back of the balloon massages the **adrenals.**
    -Relaxing the tongue releases the **vagus nerve.**

Physical stress is mismanaged dimmer switches. Short muscles compress joints, aggravating spinal disc compression and arthritis. Judgments and EmoThoughts are sources of psychological stress.

3)    Spinal Breathing:
    **-NECK**    Relaxing the throat/tongue releases neck tension.
    **-LOW BACK**   Softening the kidneys releases low back tension.

When you feel the tube and balloon, you gain access to the dimmers that control the deep muscles of the vertebra. By approaching the spine from the front, you effectively release the source of neck and lumbar tension.

# The Reboot Resets the Vagus Nerve and the Adrenals

The imagery of the Reboot is the Balloon and the Tube. I ask you to feel the back of the balloon as it inflates toward the spine and kidneys. You're also invited to open the airway by relaxing the tongue. Aiming your attention at these two anatomical areas strategically deconstructs stress and transforms trauma.

**THE TUBE  ——>  Your link to your Vagus Nerve**

Relaxing your tongue and throat opens your airway. The larger the tube is, the more easily air moves in and out of your body, making it easier to breathe. Another benefit: relaxing the tongue Reboots the vagus nerve, the dominant nerve linked with your organs.

When I introduced dimmer switches I said you have a dimmer console in your brain that manages each muscle. There's another dimmer console that controls your organs.  The vagus nerve connects to most of your organs,

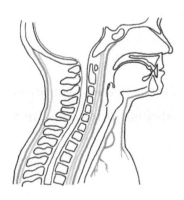

not the muscles that pull on your bones and bend your joints.  When you get upset or afraid, your vagus backfires, and your organs get tight. In many ways, tight organs reflect a deeper level of stress than muscle tension. The vagus nerve has so many branches, making it the main link to digestion, swallowing, intestinal tone, respiration, and liver function. Due to the tongue's large size and neural connections, relaxing the tongue recalibrates the vagus nerve and Reboots the visceral dimmer console, the control panel that regulates your vital organs. The vagus nerve carries the sensory data from your organs to your brain, which tells you how your body is really feeling.  Your vagus gives you your visceral truth, from your heart and your gut. This important information informs your dimmer decisions, which are then managed by the autonomic nervous system.

Like your adrenals, your vagal system either acts as though you are safe or it perceives a threat. The turtle either emerges from the shell or it retreats. Reboot Camp trained you to produce a dimmer status report and locate yourself on the adrenal spectrum. The top half of the spectrum is Foe and the lower half is Friend. Notice what your body and mind do when you are in foe mode and notice how you feel among friends. Permission is one of my favorite words because it empowers you to let go of the adrenal imperatives that keep you stressed, sick, stagnant, and stuck in your small shell.

Read about polyvagal theory to learn more. Anatomically, the vagus is a cranial nerve that emerges from the brainstem. You have a left vagus and a right vagus which exit your skull alongside the jugular veins. The vagus nerve branches out and connects to your throat, esophagus, stomach, duodenum, small intestine, and most of your large intestine. Your vagus nerve also monitors and helps regulate your lungs, heart, liver, and gallbladder too. The more thoroughly you relax your tongue and throat, the deeper you Reboot your vagal, visceral network.

**THE BALLOON   ——>   Your link to your Adrenals**

I ask you to observe your breathing balloon as it fills and empties. As you see the balloon expand in 3D, feel the back half of the balloon as it presses toward your spine. Your kidneys and your adrenal glands are located here. The word renal means kidney, and it is included in the words ad<u>renal</u> and ad<u>renal</u>ine. Nephron also means kidney, and a nephrologist is a kidney doctor. You might have heard of an Epi Pen, which is a shot of epi<u>nephrine</u>, also known as adrenaline.

Chronic adrenal activation is driven by the belief that there's a foe, a threat to your safety. Your stress level is precisely equal to the amount you believe you're in danger. You might not be in immediate danger, but when you worry, you're projecting into the future and focussing on scenarios where you're in trouble. Your cells are programmed to respond to this as if they're in immediate danger. Your belief in the bad scenario tells the cells it's real, so they act on this instruction and try to protect you. When cells perceive a threat, they increase inflammation, which is their version of the Fight response. If you're in duress, healing and repairing tissue are a low priority. Your short-term survival program diverts all your efforts toward getting safe NOW, by turning up dimmers and activating your motor system.

In contrast, when you feel your balloon massaging your kidneys, you detach from your habituated adrenal reactions. You finally stop looking for safety because you finally found it. The Reboot helps you find this safe place within yourself, building the permission to override fear. Being concerned or preoccupied are symptoms of low level fear, and when your balloon rhythmically massages your adrenals, you find permission to discharge apprehension and distractions.

The Reboot combines resetting the vagus nerve and the adrenals, clearing stress from your organs and your muscles. This simple yet comprehensive method is a powerful tool that enables you to effectively release tension globally. By recognizing the roots of the crashed loops that generate tension, you deconstruct stress. Free yourself…you're the only one who can!

We aren't figuring things out, solving problems, or rising above them. We're going through them by open the sensory side and feeling into the body. Connect to what's happening. Working with the Tube and Balloon strategically targets the roots of stress and trauma that drive dysfunction and disease. The method is to feel. Thinking doesn't Reboot anything.

Actually, EmoThinking is the flawed code that has you crashed. Feeling brings you back to reality, so you can get your bearings and gain ground.

## The Tube and the Balloon

Register your results. Like a scientist documents each experiment, notice how you feel after each mediation/treatment. Did you notice a connection between throat tension and breathing? For me personally, if I carry what I'd call the typical tension most people have in their throat, I can't really feel the back of the balloon. As soon as I relax my tongue and open the tube, I can see and feel the back of the balloon as it inflates toward my low back. Feeling the front of the balloon is relatively easy since the belly and chest expand outward during inhalation. Feeling and seeing the back half of the balloon is not as common or straightforward. The back half of the balloon the arteries and fascia behind your organs as well as the main nerves that emerge from the front of the spine.

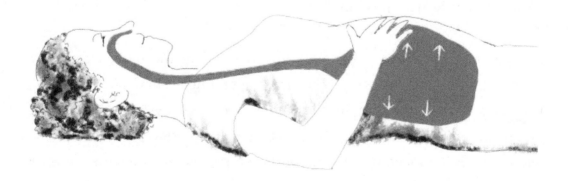

# YOUR INTRINSIC BREATH

The Reboot takes you to the lower levels of the Adrenaline Spectrum. It's simple: notice tension with your sensory side and then turn off any dimmer switches that activate your muscles. If you keep doing that, you peel away all the layers of tension until your motor system is completely unplugged. You can read about it, but to really know it, you need go inside and experience it for yourself. We can talk about dimmers all day, but you have to turn them off to know what it's like.

Free from adrenaline and thinking, your muscles lengthen. You release the physical tension that binds you and causes orthopedic pain. Another benefit of shutting off the motor system is clearing neural static. With less noise, it's quieter than ever before. Your senses are more sensitive, because they're static free. As all of this accurate data gets processed, you get a more vivid sense of what's happening, a more crisp experience. Your augmented sensory system has more bandwidth, giving you a high definition (HD) image of the moment you're in. This **Static Free** sensory upgrade improves your sensory skills, which is a major asset in your pursuit to self-heal, or heal others.

Computers have many levels, so you have to find the flawed code and rewrite it. Programs run within the larger operating system, like mac OS or Windows. If the glitch is in the larger operating system, rebooting a program won't help. The operating system is the interface, and it's how we interact with the machine. When you move the mouse, the cursor moves and registers your command. Your mind is the interface to your body; it's the neural software that controls your anatomical hardware. In the same way a person operates a computer, your mind operates you body.

Rather than focus on the superficial programs, I invite you to plunge into the base layer of your mental operating system, so you can get to the source of the issue, the root cause. If you relax completely, you arrive at the bottom of the adrenal spectrum. Your static-free senses clears your mind and restores your original, default settings. Practically speaking, this is a full Reboot. The world looks and feels different from this vantage point, and this is where you encounter your Intrinsic Breath. I choose the word *intrinsic* because it describes the inherent properties of something, and what's built-in to it.

Here, your motor system is completely off, so you're not doing anything. At the same time, your sharpened, static free senses watch your breathing balloon as it fills and empties. Whatever is happening with your balloon is happening without your involvement because you are passive and relaxed. Eventually, you realize that your body breathes by itself. You are not the one breathing, your body is doing it. Relaxing is letting go of your body, so when you let go of it completely, you're not the body that is breathing. You're the one watching and witnessing, seeing and feeling the balloon as it fills and empties. **The Intrinsic Breath is the experience of witnessing your body in its natural state, breathing all by itself.**

Shutting off dimmers and muscles gets you out of the way, and you let things unfold naturally. Your dimmers allow you to do things and change

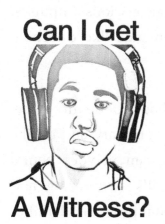

# Can I Get
# A Witness?

what happens. When you turn them off, you're no longer involved with what happens. You passively let nature take its course. Opening the sensory side allows you to become a witness, an observer. You notice tension and you release it, and then you notice more subtle tension and you let go even more, sinking down further. When you observe your balloon from this detached perspective, you become the one who sees, not the one who does.

# It All Boils Down to Safety…Reaching Home Base

Your adrenals are programmed to keep you safe by actively turning up dimmers to get you to safely. At the bottom of the Adrenal Spectrum, you're officially safe. There are no threats. You don't need to keep striving and trying to get to a safe place because you've already arrived at home base. Amazing grace! You don't need to do anything, so you don't need your muscles right now. You have the luxurious permission to let your guard down. On a more subtle level, you don't need to plan anything or think about anything. There's no need or imperative that's pulling on your attention. You don't need to be concerned about your situation. You don't need to resolve anything or prepare for something. Even your agenda to heal yourself doesn't require you to be preoccupied at this second. All of this stuff can simply sit on a shelf somewhere. The Reboot Method researches deep healing and takes you to this idyllic place where you're truly free and untethered. This chapter invites you to imagine the "adrenal-free you" and the Intrinsic Breath Meditation dares you to directly experience and embody your natural state, without the adrenal overlay.

Your survival programming has 2 main parts: identifying threats and responding to them. Once a threat is perceived, you mobilize. The sensory side is used to identify threats; the motor side responds. The mind tells the body what to do. Like light bulbs, muscles obey any dimmer signals they receive, whether they're conscious decisions or unconscious impulses. Your body will even dutifully follow useless commands like clenching your teeth when you're asleep!

The adrenals ask an important question: Friend or Foe? To identify a foe, your adrenals use your sensory awareness to keep you wary and on the lookout. Your "adrenal mind" is the survival program in your neural software that sees the world as a threat matrix. It's scrutinizing and suspicious, with paranoid tendencies. Once the adrenal program identifies a threat, it chooses a response from the 3 options it has: Freeze, Flight, or Fight. The body's dimmers and cells implement the instructions and do what the mind tells them to do.

Vigilance is helpful when you are vulnerable, but it is useless for healing. In fact, it's counterproductive and even destructive. False alarms are crashed adrenal instructions that feed disease. When the adrenal mind misidentifies threats, it sends the body on a wild goose chase toward disharmony. Even cells play along by getting inflamed and fomenting disease.

## Early Warnings

Adrenal survival programming uses the brain to run virtual scenarios to prepare for what might happen. The adrenal mind asks "what if" constantly, like a chess player thinks ahead to predict the consequences of each move. These fantasies aren't just flights of fancy; the adrenal agenda is all business. Threats need to seem real, so you'll believe there is danger. Your adrenals need you to care, so they are constantly making the case that each possible threat is real, just in case. Even if you have a misunderstanding with a friend or you are stuck in traffic, your adrenals will tell you your life is at stake, and that there is an imperative need. To the adrenal mind, every problem feels like a mortal threat.

What comes next is fascinating! Once you believe there is a foe, your adrenals have command of your attention. What do they do with your most precious resource? They generate thoughts and emotions to grapple with the foe. Your mind formulates a plan, and your body implements it. Thoughts help you decide how to respond. **Thinking is the survival software that chooses to escape, fight, or freeze.** Thinking is debating about whether to run, fight, or play dead, parsing out the 3 options it has: defend, attack, or pretend you're invisible. Chess players think through their survival options, predicting the probabilities of each possible outcome, so they can arrive at their best move.

Emotions play the vital role that links the mind to the physical body, so you respond accordingly to the perceived threat. **Emotional energy motivates the body and makes it hide, run, or fight.** Thinking helps you choose your move and emotions make sure the body follows the command and does whatever is necessary. Emotions give thoughts the traction they need to implement the decree, supplying the energy that propels the thought toward the intended outcome. Without emotion, thoughts don't usually have enough energy to generate a meaningful action.

With computers, when software processes data, it applies an algorithm and sends instructions to the hardware. The instructions need to be received and deciphered by the device so it can follow that command. To print a document, you need to tell the printer exactly where to put the ink, and which pixels get shaded. When you perceive foe, you apply the adrenal mind's algorithm and respond to the threat by activating your brain and thinking. Your adrenal mind *decides* what you'll do which dictates your motor reaction. Then, your emotions convey this command to the body so it executes the order to freeze, fight, or fly away. Emotions are the bridge that translates the brain's neural software to the body's anatomical hardware. Interestingly, the liver plays a major role in translating your emotions into actions, and we'll explore this in Book 2 of The Quantum Needle.

Gaming out scenarios to prepare for what's coming is how EmoThoughts help you survive. Squirrels are famous for working hard to store acorns, as if they are programmed or compelled. Their ability to foresee the long winter when food is scarce inspires them to stash food and diligently build their own safety net, which is quite clever. Also, if predators want to eat you, it's beneficial to be on your toes. Humans are in a different category.

Our neocortex is an advanced apparatus that imagines and envisions abstract possibilities, but it is easily co-opted by misguided survival instincts. When the glass is half empty, it perceives scarcity and the short-term logic of imminent threat. This is the *need*, the *imperative* that generates emotional reactions. When we unplug this survival program, our imagination gets repurposed We see options and choices. Our reactivity becomes creativity.

Rather than lying awake in bed with redundant EmoThoughts that make you an anxious insomniac, you could be asleep and dreaming about solutions to the challenges facing you. Your imagination can be an asset or a liability, a blessing or a curse. If you buy into your adrenal mind's foe mentality, your dream skills get hijacked, trapping you in a crashed loop. On the other hand, friendship is full of possibilities. Healing is a byproduct of collaborating with natural forces, not just surviving.

So many of us have a hard time just turning our brain off. Understanding why your adrenal mind generates EmoThoughts helps you find the switch to shut it down. Releasing the tongue and feeling the breath filling the back of the balloon are simple short cuts that help you embody safety. Reboot Camp introduces the concept of dimmer switches in your brain that control your muscles. Lifting your arm in the air is a voluntary action and turning off a dimmer switch on purpose is also your choice, a voluntary inaction. You alone command these switches, and it's your sovereign right to exert your will to the best of your ability. Turning off your EmoThinking mind is a similar choice that suspends your survival

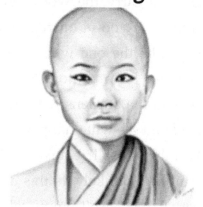

Dedicate this time
to being

Let your being be,
for the time being

program for a while. The difference is that this mental dimmer switch is deeply embedded into your Ego's Operating System, your concept of who and what you are. You'll need to step out of this crude programming that defines "the small you" so you can Reboot it, update your self-image, and reinvent yourself. You're so much more than you think!

Your operating system (OS) has many sophisticated programs that are far more creative than the simplistic options of the Freeze Flight Fight. Your physiology is a highly evolved biochemical sequence, and cells are tiny "nano bots" that follow the programs encoded in your genes. Your metabolic Qi energy is primarily derived from breathing, and your Intrinsic Breath gives you access to the source of your LifeForce. Liberating your attention from incessant thinking enables you to tap into this wellspring of energy that nature provided to you and every other living thing.

Your brain is an astonishingly advanced, multilayered network imbued with Artificial Intelligence. Given its complexity, it often needs updates, servicing, and repair. To reboot a device you must stop using it and drain the circuits. I'll repeat this crucial fact: you must stop using it for a while. That means: no thinking or emoting for the time being!

Do you carry the world on your shoulders? If you falter, will people suffer? If you're unwell, your own health keeps your hands full, so you might be the one who suffers. It's true that there's an endless need and demand for attention. Yet nature gave you your shoulders, and it also created the burdens that weigh them down. For a few moments, drop the load and see what happens. That's what this experiment is designed to test. Will the sky fall? Unlikely. Will anyone suffer if you relax deeply for a few minutes? Unlikely. Is this a safe experiment? That's for you to answer. A verbal "yes" isn't empirical data, and predictions aren't evidence. You've got to run this scenario of radical release and Reboot fully to see what the results will be.

# Judgments and Assessments

Judgments have a strong emotional component whereas assessments provide feedback in a more neutral way. Judging your breath as shallow causes you to react by taking a deep breath. Rather than remain in the sensory side to observe what's happening, you activate the motor system and turn up dimmers. This derails your Reboot.

The judgment of shallowness includes an emotion that translates to: "my breath is flawed and bad." The emotion activates a physical response and compels you to do something right away. You reflexively try to compensate by jumping into action. It seems like it's your will, because you huff and puff and you do it on purpose. You're motivated to intervene and convert your shallow breath into something better, yet your ambition to fix your flawed breathing has you reacting to your survival impulses and chasing your tail.

The assessment of shallowness has much less emotion than the judgment of shallowness. Without this emotional charge, you're not compelled to react. You're not in a critical state, so you don't need to intervene. After all, you've been breathing since birth, successfully enough to survive. You can stay with your sensory side and feel what your shallow breath feels like. Give yourself permission to be with the tension. Once you stop resisting it, you can feel it and map it out. Soon enough, you'll find the dimmers you left on and turn them down. This is the difference between Rebooting and reacting.

It's true that we often breathe shallowly, so becoming aware of it is good. We'll use this information to diagnose our dimmer console and release our background tension. Rather than override your breathing rhythm, pay attention to what's going on and learn something. Judging the breath as flawed isn't mindfulness, it's just another crashed EmoThought loop. Like

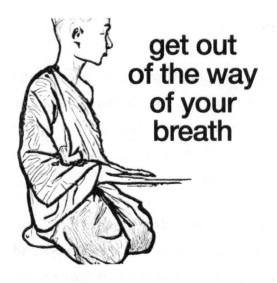

**get out of the way of your breath**

physical discomfort and pain, EmoThoughts activate the motor side and compel a reaction, moving you up the adrenal spectrum. When you judge your breath as shallow, you're a bad breather! When you diligently do your techniques, you compensate and make amends, becoming a good breather. Either way, you're trapped by judgments, and the body is either stifled with tension or micromanaged with techniques. Put these loops down and settle into the fact that you're an Intrinsic Breather!

## The Intrinsic Breath = No Tension + No Technique

Tension is neglect, and technique is micromanaging. The Intrinsic Breath is the middle path, the juxtaposition of being fully connected, yet totally detached. The sensory side is open and the motor is off. Neglect is unconscious, and micromanaging is hyperaware. The trick is to hold your attention steady, so you can connect and also get out of the way. It's a big ask, so consider this an open invitation to find your center.

Turning the motor side off includes reducing background tension AND declining trying to help by using techniques. Tension and technique are the 2 big obstacles that keep the motor side running and prevent Step 1 of the Reboot. Relaxing means unplugging the reactive adrenal mind. Tension and technique are both motivated by judgments and EmoThoughts, so when you quell your overactive adrenals you remove both obstacles, paving your path to healing.

Our background tension is the result of leaving dimmers on constantly. Once we acclimate to tight muscles, we habituate to our not-so-new-normal stress level. Reboot Camp cited pain and adrenaline as the two reasons muscles tighten. When the brain deciphers pain, it automatically turns up dimmers. Adrenaline also stimulates contractions in overt and covert ways. Fighting and running away require amping up the motor side. The Freeze response is more subtle, because we don't physically move. Frozen adrenal energy activates the adrenal mind, which runs scenarios and generates the EmoThoughts that compel the body to remain vigilant.

People in Freeze mode are active even when they are physically still because their body is experiencing and living out the virtual scenarios in their mind. They are occupied internally, contending with moments that seem real, but aren't. Being preoccupied is actually a mildly frozen state, describing the slippery slope of EmoThoughts that crash toward higher stress and the deep freeze. Anxiety converts daydreams into daymares, and a panic attack is a nightmare while you're awake. Freeze is the inward implosion of attention, and most of us have adapted to living with a moderate degree of frozen preoccupation. Many asymptomatic people who function and live normal lives are cloaked with a veil of dissociation and disconnect. Certain parts of them remain unconscious. The background tension in our bodies stems from pain and the subliminal EmoThoughts persistently droning in the back of our minds.

Technique is our reaction to being frozen. It's our attempt to snap out of being self consumed and lost in thought. When you recognize you're stuck, you want to do something to get free. Doing something leads you to the motor side, so you turn up dimmers. The trouble is, your dimmers are already too high because you left them on unconsciously. Shallow breathing is usually the result of unconscious background tension in the throat and torso. **Technique doesn't fix tension, relaxing does.** At any moment, you can turn your dimmers down!

Don't take the bait and activate! Stay with the sensory side and feel your semi-frozen state. Your new job is to notice when you get tempted to do something. Decline the impulse to force air; open the breathing tube instead. Feel the back of the breathing balloon as it inflates toward your spine, kidneys, and adrenals. Your EmoThoughts supply the rationale (thoughts) and the motivation (emotional motive) to activate your motor side. It's very easy to slip into judgment, and as soon as you do, your assessments get distorted into judgments which becomes reactions.

Rebooting requires deep discipline, keeping your attention on the sensory side. If self-healing was easy, I wouldn't need to treat patients or write this. On a daily basis, I use my sensory side to activate my patient's sensory side. This is where the medicine is, not in *doing*. When I palpate a patient's tissues, I feel my way through the fibers to the restriction. Once I connect, my hands move a little, but I'm not really doing anything. I'm following their body, which provides the feedback the body needs to work itself out. The more keenly I connect in real time, the better the results. Listen to your symptoms, your pain, and your EmoThoughts. Be with them, without judgment. Stay with the sensory side, and be present, so they can resolve the glitch and Reboot their crashed code. It's simple, but not always easy.

Releasing your background tension and thawing out is a huge relief. When dimmers are high, muscles are short, making it harder for the balloon to expand and fill. This physical tension in the torso restricts the range of motion of the diaphragm and lungs, making the breath smaller. Shutting off all dimmers and completely relaxing lengthens each muscle. It feels like taking off a corset or a tight, restrictive wetsuit. Your breath suddenly becomes effortless. Once you experience the logic of release, you see how trying isn't the solution. Trying stems from the adrenal imperative of need, and it's just another aspect of the same crashed loops. Surrendering softens struggling and suffering. Relaxing resolves rigidity and removes restrictions.

# Technique is Folly

Attempting to breathe better is a reaction, which is a primitive response. Reactions are reflexes, a "knee-jerk" type of lower level response to a stimulus. Our animal instincts of survival are deep programs that instruct us to get safe. Fear accelerates this urge to get safe, which compels us to try and get safe NOW! If we don't reflexively react, we stay aligned with the long-term vision and the natural flow of things. Reacting is short-term logic that's unaware of the big picture. Neurologically, a reaction comes from the brain stem and reptilian brain, which I call the adrenal mind. A crafted response passes through the neocortex, the more evolved network that allows us to formulate abstract ideas, language, and the dream skills that conjure up scenarios.

If you summon your will and decide to stop EmoThinking, you awaken an even higher level response that comes directly from the heart, not the brain. This part of you sees beyond the push/pull that your adrenal mind creates as it bounces from judgment to judgment. The brain processes data, and it's full of opinions, making it hot and cold. The heart holds a steady rhythm and has the humility to witness.

### Taoist Drivers Don't Swerve

When a teenager learns to drive, they typically turn abruptly and oversteer. As they veer off course, they realize they need to turn the other way to correct, and they overdo that too. Once they oversteer, they end up swerving again trying to compensate. This cycle has them reacting to their reaction.

Once they get the feel of how the car moves, they can just lightly turn the wheel and carve a smooth path. No longer reacting, they employ a measured response. When they can be relaxed and sit behind the wheel of the moving car, they're ready to drive safely. We think that learning how to drive is about controlling the car, but it's really about controlling yourself. Learning to drive is really *feeling safe while driving*. You are safe when you are in control of yourself and your adrenal reactions. If you don't feel safe, you overreact, and the car overreacts too.

Novice drivers need to get the feel of how the car moves, and novice breathers need to get the feel of how their body breathes. Let go of trying to breathe, and sit in the passenger seat. Let your body drive. Your respiration is a self driving car equipped with highly evolved BioTechnology. Your body breathes by itself when you're asleep, so you're often on autopilot. You can take manual control of your breath at any time, but why not let your body drive? After all, your automated breath automatically activates and animates your anatomy. Your breath has carried you since birth, and your mother's breath oxygenated your cells in utero. I'm inviting you to trust nature to sustain you while you listen to the 13 minute Intrinsic Breath Meditation. Let's test the hypothesis that nature built your body, and nature also maintains it. The current of the lazy river will carry you…

Your Intrinsic Breath is the source of your LifeForce, the wellspring that generates your metabolic Qi. If you want to improve your condition, tap your Intrinsic Breath and channel this resource into your organs, tissues, and body systems. The more you get out of the way of your breath, the more directly you connect with your essence. Once you accept the fact that your body breathes by itself, you stop trying to re-invent the wheel. Instead, use the fact that wheels roll to gracefully propel your vessel forward.

—    Listen to Intrinsic Breath Meditation Audio    —

# THE THREE PRINCIPLES

The 3 Principles are how we process things. It's a 3 stage process in which you let the moment in, you process it, and then you release it. At any moment, you can *Apply The Principles*. It's as easy as 1, 2, 3.

## Accept

## Feel

## Release

Step 1: **Accept** = Allow reality to be what it is. Let it in.
Step 2: **Feel** = Experience the moment you're in. Process it.
Step 3: **Release** = Detach. Let it go.

## The 3 Principles are....

### The Algorithm

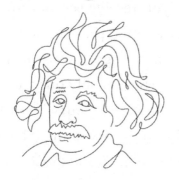

### Of Health

### The 3 Phases

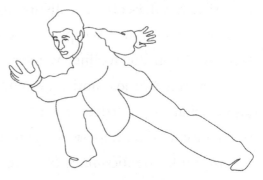

### Of Flow

# First: Accept

Acceptance is first, otherwise we block reality. In math, the most basic equation is $x=x$. We can translate this into plain English with the common phrase "it is what it is." We call $x$ a *variable* because it can be any number. It's just a place-holder that marks the space and holds the position, so the content doesn't matter. Every moment, each NOW, is a new $x$, a blank moment in time that you'll occupy very soon. **Each "$x$" is an experience that you have**. Any given moment can be filled with good sensations or pain, your breath could be easy and free, or it could be shallow. You go up and down the adrenal spectrum, and you experience many moments, some positive and some negative.

Regardless of the sensations you are feeling, if you judge them and wish they were different, you are out of touch with *what is*. Whatever this moment gives you, whatever you plug in for $x$, you'll end up with $x=x$. Even when x is negative and something you don't want, $-x$ is still $-x$. Wishing $x$ isn't $x$ refutes this most basic truth, so Acceptance is first.

# Second: Feel

Once you Accept that it is what it is, you can dial into *what it is*. Process it. Experience it. Discern and distinguish it. When you receive sensory input and you let it all in (Accept), you connect directly to the present moment. Whatever you are feeling, whether you like it or not: go toward it, not away from it. Witness and experience your NOW. There is only one way to know what any particular $x$ is: investigate and immerse yourself in the moment you're in. Experience your present reality fully. Accepting (Step 1) opens you to the incoming content, so you can hone in on the exact value of this particular $x$, and Feel it fully (Step 2).

As you develop your sensory skills, you increase your accuracy. When we measure things and quantify them, we can use more decimal places to describe any number more precisely. A number like 2.71828… is more precise than the truncated version of 2.7. We can also round this number up to 3 which is simpler, but less accurate. Approaching the incoming moment openly and applying your attention to your static-free sensory signals provides detailed and precise incoming information. You connect to the intrinsic truth and experience the totality of whatever this moment brings.

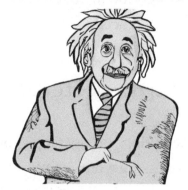

**Mathematicians**

**Make It Count**

Feeling is my primary tool when working with patients. My ability to get clear and relevant information from my patient's body and mind improves my ability to help them. I don't apply techniques to my patients: I cut through neural static and listen to their body. Once engaged, it responds, and I follow the tissue and do whatever it wants. It leads the way, and I encourage the release. The more I open myself to all the content they are expressing, the better the results. Feeling makes me more useful.

Information comes in many forms, and the next book explores the many languages your body and mind use to communicate with itself. Feeling is how you register all sensations, thoughts, emotions, and ideas you have. It's everything you experience. Feeling *into* yourself connects you to what's actually happening, connecting you to what is. Every scientific discovery must be grounded in truth, so that the equations add up and match reality. Precise Feeling gives you this solid foundation.

As you work with the Reboot and release your chronic tension, you start to recognize your patterns, your crashed loops. The fog of neural static clears away and you gain acuity. You get more concise information from your own body when you are lower down on the Adrenal Spectrum. Once connected to your internal environment, you can see clearly. Feeling allows you to determine what's real and what's noise and fiction. You have to sift through the mental haze of EmoThoughts to get to the pertinent data, the stuff you need.

# Third: Release

Accepting is opening yourself to the incoming moment. Feeling is processing your NOW. Once you immerse yourself in your experience, Release it. Let go of it and detach. The moment comes and then it goes. Let it go. Accepting is the first principle because it allows you to receive what's coming, and Release is last because it acknowledges that time is moving. If you hold on to the outgoing moment, you are tethered to the past and resisting the flow of time. The more you focus on the past, the more you aren't Accepting the incoming moment. Before you know it, you revert back to wishing $x$ does not equal $x$.

$X$ is always a variable, so it changes with each new NOW. The equation $x=x$ is remarkably fluid because our conditions are constantly changing. It's a new equation every moment, a new set of circumstances. Linear time is the string of unique moments that all line up. If we are to keep our wits and navigate through this ever-changing world, we need to reapply the Principles often, so we can Accept and Feel whatever life throws at us. Release takes you full circle, so can to reapply the Principles and Accept what's coming in. As you train with the Reboot and the Intrinsic Breath, you gain the ability to Accept Feel Release. Each time you cycle through all three phases, you get more connected to your static-free reality.

Letting go empties you out and allows you to Accept the new moment that's coming. Each new moment presents you with new conditions to

Accept, something new to recognize and Feel. If you let go of that experience, you can greet the next new moment with openness. Japanese Zen Buddhism has a concept called Beginner's Mind, which is being completely open to whatever the moment offers. This profound Acceptance to the Now requires you to Release any influence from the past or the future. When you reapply the 3 Principles, you realize that **Release gives you permission to Accept**.

The more frequently you complete all 3 Principles, the more you allow moments to pass through you. Being in this flow generates your presence, which quantifies how much of you is here in reality. Otherwise, past moments clog up your Qi Machine and you aren't really here, now. If you don't Release, you get stuck in delusion, because that past moment is gone, and it is not real any more. You end up ignoring or blocking the new moment, and you don't connect to what is happening in the moment you're in. This oversight is costly because this HereNow is your only reality. As soon as you squeeze and try to grasp onto your experience, you get stuck at the 3rd Principle and refuse to Release. The flow is blocked and you stagnate. Getting sucked into good memories or past trauma is way too easy, which makes it really hard to attain enlightenment.

We also get drawn into wishing for a brighter tomorrow or prophesying a catastrophic future. If you look forward to a better time or you dread impending events, you are running a virtual scenario about the future and your attention isn't HereNow. These past reflections and future projections are just shadows on the wall. When your attention is on what was or what will be, you can't connect to what is. If your adrenals are barking in your brain causing you to think and emote, a part of you is frozen and locked in a crashed loop. Wherever this part of you is, it is trapped in a time warp and exiled from the real world. When these lost parts of you Reboot, they get reintegrated. Unprocessed moments finally get processed when they are Accepted and Felt. Applying the 3rd Principle of Release clears them

75

from your system, cleansing old wounds and trauma. The Reboot Method helps you finally process your backlog, so you become more nimble. Book 2 of The Quantum Needle isn't strictly about self-healing, it's about being present.

Each experience is a unique snowflake in the relentless blizzard of time. This constant flurry of moments just keeps going. Recognize when you check out and retreat into your EmoThinking adrenal mind, your small self. This helps you Accept the fact that a part of you isn't here. Don't let your mindfulness get derailed from judgments. Even if you are tight and frozen, you can witness what is happening. If you judge yourself or if you are trying, you didn't let go yet. Judging is a reaction that activates your motor side and turns up dimmers in an effort to change what's happening. You end up fighting what is. As you work with the 3 Principles, you come to understand that Release dovetails into Acceptance and that letting go is the best way to open up. This is when you feel the flow that the Taoists talk about. In this new moment, perhaps more of you is here, and you can recognize what that feels like. It might feel better. Whether you are attracted to this moment or repulsed by it, you can Accept it, Feel it, and Release that too.

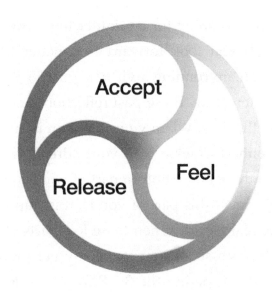

# Unpacking Your Adrenals: Healing Trauma

The 3 Principles of Accept Feel Release are how health works, and the 3F's of Freeze Flight Fight are how disease works. They're mirror images of each other!

## 1. Freeze is Non-Acceptance
## 2. Flight is Non-Feeling
## 3. Fight is Non-Release

The 3 Principles describe flow, the functional feedback loop of health and the 3F's are the adrenal crashed loop of disease. I hope to illustrate many valuable truths to you, and this might be the most important implication of the 3 Principles of the Reboot Method. Are you ready to see your healthy side AND your dysfunctional, broken parts?

Your diagnosis identifies where your issue is, To heal, you need to find out where you're stuck. Once you recognize whether you are in Freeze, Flight, or Fight mode, you can apply the Principle that gets you back on track. This rewrites that flawed code and Reboots the glitch that derailed your nervous system. Applying all 3 Principles restores flow to your Qi Machine, so you optimize your potential and live your best life.

**Freeze** is when we can't or won't Accept what's happening. We dissociate, and part of us denies the reality we can't accept. **Freeze is trauma**, the breaking point where we buckle under the stress. Flight and fight are stressful, but not traumatic. When in shock, the nervous system is overwhelmed with too much electricity and unable to function, so that moment remains unprocessed. When we don't Accept a moment, we fragment ourself and create a region within ourself to put the event we can't deal with. The mind gets split into two parts, creating a partition in our mental hard drive. We build a wall and put that experience behind it, stored somewhere in the BodyMind. We bury it and try to forget about it, pretending it never happened, but the problem with full denial is that it's not true. Nature always wins because $x = x$ regardless.

Because Freeze puts us out of touch with reality, it has costly consequences. The part of us that actually lived through the traumatic event is trapped on the other side of the wall. When we compart*mentalize*, our wounded parts are exiled in our subconscious and stored in the body's tissues. Part of us is missing, lost in the mental maze we built to insulate ourselves. We have blind spots, and when big chunks of us disappear, we become hollow. The Harry Potter stories include a magical "cloak of invisibility" that hides whatever is underneath it. In a similar way, Freeze magically hides trauma.

**Flight** is when we Accept the moment but we don't Feel it, so we retreat from the experience. We are open enough to Accept reality, so we are whole and unbroken, yet we're unwilling to stay with it and actually be there. We can evacuate to escape the threat, or we can knuckle down and block it. Flight insulates us from Feeling, by avoiding or repelling what's happening. Rather than run away, a shield helps us deflect threats. We can't outrun arrows, so a shield gives us a safe zone, a bunker to hide behind. We retreat into our shell and thicken our skin, making armor. The Freeze response builds walls *within* ourselves while Flight builds walls *around* ourselves. Both defensive strategies protect us from a hostile environment.

Flight is often subtle, like changing the subject to avoid talking about something uncomfortable.

**Fight** is when we resist what is, and we try to change things. We've Accepted and Felt something, but our attempt to intervene becomes counterproductive when we force it. We might even want to be helpful, but our efforts end up backfiring because we try too hard. The good news is we're no longer frozen and helpless. We're also not defensive, hiding behind a shield or looking for an exit. We turn and face the threat, and we're invested in seeing it through. We're willing to claim our space and eradicate any threat, which is progress. Fight is when the victim stands up for themselves and pushes back on the threat, like a desperate, cornered animal. Fight is a necessary phase toward claiming power, but there is a flaw to the fight impulse: it is a *reaction to being powerless before*. Often beneath the anger, there is sadness and grief. Underneath the hard shell is a soft and squishy interior. Fighting is still tied to being a victim, so a fighter is really a sheep dressed in wolf's clothing.

**Accept**  =  Show up  —>  No walls. Thaw, AntiFreeze

**Feel**    =  Stand in  —>  Uninsulated, full experience

**Release** =  Move on  —>  Detach, let go, forgive

| Principle | Adrenal | Tool | Blockage |
|---|---|---|---|
| 1. Accept | Freeze | Invisibility | Inputs |
| 2. Feel | Flight | Shield | Processor |
| 3. Release | Fight | Sword | Outputs |

# The 3 Principles Debunks "Taking a Deep Breath"

The Intrinsic Breath is your natural state, where you breathe freely, with no tension and no technique! Reflexively taking a deep breath is a reaction to the judgment of shallowness, which derails the 3 Principles. We don't Accept the shallowness, we don't Feel the shallowness, and we don't Release it either. In general, the unconscious background tension in our bodies is a product of the Freeze response: EmoThinking is dissociative, an imaginary fantasy world cut off from reality. We don't even know we're tight because we've habituated to it. We're unaware, oblivious, checked out, vacant, and uncomfortably numb!

Being mindful and paying attention is our attempt to show up and Accept the moment we're in. We successfully met the 1st Principle by thawing out enough to become aware of our body and how it's breathing. Then, we immediately run for cover. Rather than stand in and Feel, we judge our breath as shallow and jump into action. We avoid Feeling by hiding behind the shield of our opinions, the mental armor that insulates us.

**Taking a deep breath is the Fight response**, using technique to change what's happening. We unfroze for a second and we didn't like what we saw, so rather than Feel the shallowness, we attack it instead. We try to override the shallowness by forcing air. Our attempt to self-correct is just another compensation, a defensive overreaction, like our teenage driver swerving. Our mindful moment gets co-opted by judgments which oscillate between ignoring our breath (Freeze) and micromanaging it (Fight). The remedy is to Feel, and be with it. As soon as you notice yourself wanting to change something, recognize that you are resisting, and fighting *what is*. Apply the 3rd Principle of Release. Most people aren't readyarrive at Release, you might need to go back to the beginning: Accept and Feel whatever is bugging you.

# What is False Detachment?

Like numbers and the alphabet, the 3 Principles are in order, so you must complete them in order. You have to Accept and Feel something before you can Release it. You've got to attach before you detach. You've got to connect before you disconnect. You've got to hold on to something before you can let it go. To even get to the 3rd Principle, you have to Accept and Feel, without judgment. Only then can you attempt the final task and truly let go of it.

When you try to Release too early, you're just avoiding something unpleasant. You're stuck on the 2nd Principle, using the Flight Response to avoid Feeling. This shortcut doesn't get you anywhere. There's a ton of false detachment, where people think they let go of old wounds. If you Release before you Feel, you're only letting go of the mental version, your projections of what happened. The bulk of the content gets stored as trapped emotional energy in the organs and in your nervous system, exiled in the frozen basement within your BodyMind. You can let go of the cognitive part of what happened, but your system still holds the stagnant Qi energy that wasn't fully processed.

Do yourself a favor and stop *trying* to Release. You can't force yourself to let go, just like you can't force yourself to shut off a dimmer. Once you notice your tension without judging it, you can effectively relax. Rather than EmoThinking and remaining helpless, go back to the beginning and Accept whatever is bugging you. Then Feel the feelings of that moment somatically in your body. When you immerse yourself, and attach to your experience, you'll be tempted to hold on and identify with what happened. Release is so hard because you must let go of what is deeply personal and familiar. True detachment is only attained when you complete the cycle of Accept Feel Release, which means unconditional Acceptance, Feeling deeply, and radical Release.

# Healing Converts Freeze, Flight, Fight into Accept, Feel, Release

**What is Trauma?**

The mind's primary task is to perceive what is happening, so it can arrive at the best response to the current situation. We need an accurate "sensory status report" so we can deduce a creative, motor solution to the challenges we face. To meet the moment, we must face the facts. Accepting *what is* connects us with reality, so we can eventually find the best path forward.

When overwhelmed, the nervous system is overloaded with too much current. This surge of electricity turns up every dimmer switch and literally shocks the tissues and organs, scorching the body's anatomical hardware. When this lightning bolt hits the brain, the tiny wires that conduct signals through the mind's neural software get overheated, damaging and traumatizing these subtle circuits. If the mind gets fried, it is rendered incapable of functioning. The sensory side is not able to perceive what is happening, so we become dissociated from reality. We become isolated from others and alienated to the world around us. This extreme blast is Icy Hot, overheating the system while sending a chill through the spine.

When we don't show up because we shut down, our frozen parts are suspended. Shock traumatizes us and prevents us from Accepting what's happening. Due to the extreme neural static, we can't receive the incoming sensory data, let alone process it. The moment, the *"x"* of HereNow, doesn't just evaporate and disappear, it gets stored in our subconscious mind and in our body. It will remain below conscious awareness until we dare Accept the fact that it happened. Thawing out takes your cryogenically preserved content out of the deep freeze. Freeze checks out; Acceptance checks in.

Freeze is why and how we suppress traumatic experiences, rejecting them to avoid dealing with what happened. Like everything adrenal, it's a way to insulate us from a harsh reality. The Freeze response empowers our ego to take drastic measures to keep us safe, by storing traumatic events behind a wall that it builds in the mind. It knowingly blocks us from processing the event, supposedly for our own good. Since we store these intense experience and suppress them on purpose, why does trauma resurface? Why do people dream about traumatic events? Why do we remember? Why do we conjure up the past and relive it? The answer is: WE'RE TRYING TO PROCESS IT.

Denying these past moments actually anchors you to them. Trauma haunts people because the system is attempting to bring the truth of what happened into the light. Evolution demands that you become aware and experience the moments of your life. Some part of you is dissatisfied with checking out, and this part of you compels you to face it. It seems like a curse to be haunted by the past, but your system is trying to clear itself. Pain tells you about an issue with your body, like a built-in self-diagnostic mechanism. Your mind has a similar way to alert you about problems with your software: they're called EmoThoughts. If you examine your EmoThoughts and self-talk, you'll see the skeletons in your closet. They are your ghosts with unresolved business, trapped in the limbo between the dark, subliminal cellar and the conscious light of day.

One way or another, all unresolved experiences will knock at your door and tug at your attention. They'll ferment and rumble around in your subconscious and they'll bubble up to the surface as physical disease or mental imbalance. Like a volcano spewing lava, your system will try to relieve the pressure. It can be a violent eruption or a slow venting. It can be obvious for others to see, or it can all happen inside you, hidden from view. When you Freeze, you pretend to fool yourself. Since you can't fool Mother Nature, and you're a product of nature, you can't really fool yourself. You

83

can distract yourself, but you'll tend to gravitate toward the blocks. Your system recognizes that your mental hard drive has a partition, so it wants to address your crashed loops and be whole.

**Transforming Trauma**

Past events won't stop haunting you until you apply all 3 Principles and actually process them cleanly. It's not easy, and there are 3 big requirements: Accept what happened, Feel and experience that moment fully, Release it all. Even if you think you did it already, open yourself yet again. Feel what's cooking inside you. After immersing yourself in that moment and attaching to that experience, let go of it. Release it and detach. Move on. Don't linger or look back. Look ahead and look inwardly: Accept your incoming Now! Your health may well depend on it.

The first step toward resolving trauma is Acceptance, which takes down the walls and lets the data arrive at the processor. The 2nd Principle is to open your processor and truly experience the moment you're in. The Flight response insulates you by minimizing Feeling, like dipping your toe in the water or having one foot out the door. Flight glosses over it and calls it complete. You froze because you were overwhelmed. As you thaw out, you'll need to give yourself permission to open your heart, dive into your NOW, and immerse yourself. You went to all the trouble to build walls within yourself to segregate this traumatic moment because it seemed like an existential threat, a threat to your existence. Affirm that you are safe now, and that the past can't hurt you anymore. Drop your shield, stand in, and dare to Feel.

Like any adrenal strategy, Freeze and Flight are only useful in the short term. You can pretend to not see and you can suspend disbelief for a while, but you can't sustain it. Reality always wins because $x$ is always $x$. Freeze can never be an effective defense because part of you knows that you're just trying to insulate yourself from the harsh reality you're ignoring. Freeze builds walls within the self and your ego convinces you there is nothing stored on the other side. In contrast, Flight isn't oblivious or in full denial because you Accept the fact those feelings exist, but you avoid Feeling the ones you don't like. Freeze believes there is nothing hidden away, while Flight knows there is something in the basement, but is unwilling to look.

I can't judge whether it is safe for you to unearth whatever you've buried. Instead, I invite you to ask yourself if you are ready to absorb those moments. Most people become aware of things in stages, processing one layer at a time, in bite-sized pieces. There is an interesting dynamic between the part of you that wants to remain unconscious and the part that wants to become conscious. Sit with these two parts of yourself and soften. Get grounded. Apply the 3 Principles. Open the tube and feel the back of the balloon. Trust that you will find your path to resolution. It might take longer than you prefer, but it will happen in due time!

If you do open your pandora's box, and you dare to Feel deeply, please apply the 3rd Principle and Release it. Don't linger in your wounds or indulge your emotions. It is very easy to wallow in "woe is me" and get entangled with the victim persona. Nature can be cruel and perhaps you suffered an injustice. Most of us have been on the short end of the stick and hurt by the world at some point. If you **identify with your wound**, you attach yourself to it and refuse to let it go. *Wound Worshippers* are stuck at the 3rd Principle, unwilling to complete the process and let go. They hold on to the past and use it to define who they are, so their shield becomes a disfigured badge of honor. Trapped in Feel, they relive the past, doomed to repeat history rather than learn from it and evolve. Fighting tries to change things that already happened. Fighters are grappling with what was, and trying to change what is. Fighters can't Accept or Feel their own truth, so they stagnate and stew in their own judgmental juices.

Compared to Freeze and Flight, the Fight response is progress because you turn and face the problem. But rather than letting it be, fighting urges you to react and apply a counter-force. You swim upstream and fight the flow of time, resisting reality. When you come to terms and make peace with your past, you drop your sword and Release what was. You forgive everyone involved and your deep compassion allows you to heal. Now that you understand how the 3 Principles and the 3F's reflect each other, you can Accept what comes out of the box, Feel the hurt or the joy, and then Release that experience entirely.

## Personal Power

The Three Principles help you reclaim your personal power. A traumatized person in Freeze Mode is entirely helpless. The internal mechanisms that generate self-esteem are broken so the person has no access to their core energy, their source. *Flighters* are whole and unbroken internally, but stuck playing defense, wanting to escape to get somewhere safe. They have enough power to run away, or retreat inwardly behind shields and fences, but they are not powerful enough to claim space. Fight is a step toward claiming space, but fighters are desperately trying to avoid being powerless, groping for power rather than actually being powerful. Fighters might temporarily reclaim turf, but fighters can't authentically *occupy* space.

Fighters are powerful enough to attack and perpetrate, but they are unable to create. Using power to attack others, or yourself, just creates more victims. When cornered, defensive victims eventually fight back, lash out, and attack. Getting stuck in the Fight Response traps them in "an eye for an eye" mentality, which feeds the karmic loop of suffering. This cycle is truly vicious. For fighters, surrender is not an option and letting go seems toxic. Yet the 3rd Principle is Release, detach. You don't have to condone what happened, but time compels you to concede that it did happen, forgive everyone involved, and move forward. Accept the incoming moment and apply the 3 Principles. Otherwise, your EmoThoughts endlessly litigate everything.

Inside each fighter is a powerless victim. Their aggression is a reaction to feeling powerless (Frozen) or weak (Flight). If you Accept and Feel your vulnerability and weakness, you will be able to Release it and Reboot that broken circuit. Releasing your wounded persona connects you to the wellspring of your true power. Moving on is really moving through, which puts you in the flow. Letting go is the final step that liberates you from reacting to what was. Deeply commune with what is, and then Release it. The more frequently you apply the 3 Principles, the more you raise your frequency. Resolving the resistance of Fight unveils the truth that peace is the path of power.

# Notes from My Clinic

I've treated hundreds of patients who told me they already processed their trauma through therapy. Ironically, as I hold their tissue in my hands, I often feel the many layers that were not processed. They healed on a cognitive level, but many somatic lessons remained unprocessed. When I touch a person's liver, kidney, esophagus, gut, brain, vagus nerve, or ankle, I immediately tune into what's wrong and I connect to the wounded part. Crashed tissues are repeating an automated reaction. I trace this discord up into the part of the brain that has also crashed. I map out their body and chart out the regions they inhabit and the parts that remain unoccupied, unexplored, or unembodied.

Inserting acupuncture needles and manually listening into tissues activates a response in the brain. It realizes I'm there and that I'm connected to this glitch. This opens up whatever is stored in the tissue and shielded from the brain. If the injury carries a strong emotional charge, the brain pulls up the unprocessed energy from storage and takes it out of the subconscious basement. This first step of Acceptance removes the walls that blocks conscious awareness. Once the mind Accepts the content that was stored in the body's somatic cellar, it can Feel it and ultimately Release it.

Holding my attention steady and remaining connected to the tissue and the brain provides realtime empathy so the body and mind can processes this difficult experience. I stay right there with it while it works out the issue and I don't get enmeshed with it. My role is to create a safe container that allows the entire system to Feel all aspects of itself. Once it processes whatever it just unEarthed, I coax Release. When the brain and body reconnect, I stop treating and I let the system reintegrate. If I linger, I end up micromanaging and overloading the patient's nervous system. I trust that it will reintegrate this frozen wound in due time. I see patients once or twice a month to allow enough time for the brain and the body to process the content and reintegrate. My treatments mediate a conversation between the tissue and the brain. This dialogue harmonizes the body with the mind, giving the anatomical hardware better instructions. Neural software also benefits from the updates it receives from the soma. The basis of medicine is the recognition of what is, which requires the humility to bear witness.

Your meditations are your treatments and reading this book is like studying a medical textbook. Self-healing is not always easy because it requires devotion, diligence, and persistent practice. At any moment, Feel your breathing balloon and notice your dimmer status. What's your body up to and how's your EmoThinking mind doing? It's always a good time to check in. Bravely approach yourself mindfully, and Accept Feel Release whatever you encounter. The odds are you'll get derailed. When you do, you can always go to your sensory side and Accept what is. As you keep Accepting, you begin to Feel. If you keep up and stay engaged, you'll probably attach to whatever is happening and you'll resist letting go. That's your cue to detach, and trust Release. Remember that if you don't

Release, you can't Accept, which slows your flow and diminishes your capacity to accrue power and execute your will. It's seems odd at first, but letting go actually gives you more control. The upcoming chapter is laser-focused on building enough trust, so you finally need have the permission to let it all go.

The 3 Principles of the Reboot Method set up ideal conditions where you mediate your inner conflicts. At any moment, repeat the mantra of Accept Feel Release. Give yourself permission to trust your flow. Dare to Accept and Feel, knowing that you'll soon Release it. This clears any glitches that clog up your processor and dampen your Qi Machine. Even though I work with my hands, my entire body feels what is going on. I ask you to embody the understanding, and venture deeper into your experiential networks. If you want better results and profound changes, take an adrenal trust fall.

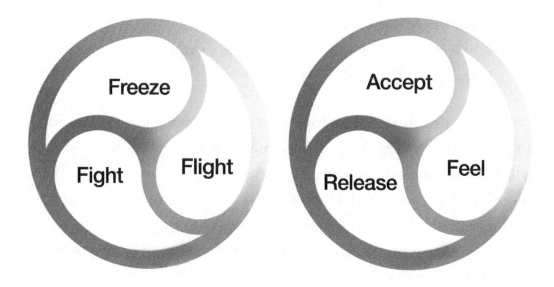

Rebooting converts
Vicious Cycles into Compassion Cycles

Freeze

Fight    Flight

Accept

Release    Feel

# The Trust Falls of Relaxation

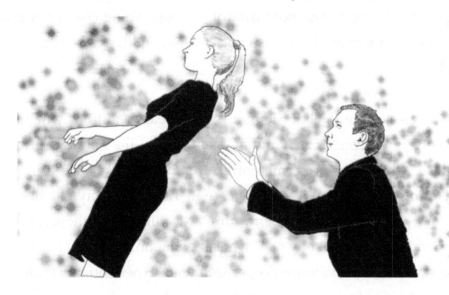

Reboot Camp invites you to turn off your dimmers, unplug your motor side, and relax all the way…down to the bottom of the Adrenal Spectrum. The Balloon and Tube imagery connects you to your adrenals and your vagus nerve, so you can release deeply. The Reboot Meditation culminates with turning off the master dimmer. After this, I mention 2 more ideas:

-You might notice that your body breathes by itself.

    The Intrinsic Breath: Chapter 1

-You might feel heavy, as if gravity suddenly got stronger.

    Relaxing is a Trust Fall: Chapter 3

The Intrinsic Breath and these Trust Falls of Relaxation map out the terrain at the lower end of the Adrenal Spectrum. When you stop reacting, your static-free sensory side awakens and sees what's really going on. When you're grounded, you get clear insights that catalyze profound experiences, creating tectonic shifts that transform you. Two important implications of the Reboot: your Intrinsic Breath is automated and *muscles are anti-gravity devices*. I asked you to let go of your breath; now I'm inviting you to let go of your body and your bones!

A full Reboot is when your motor system is totally off, and your sensory side is wide open. The Intrinsic Breath is the experience of being totally passive while you witness your body breathing without your help. You're not the one breathing, you're the witness, the one watching and feeling your body breathe. Another byproduct and consequence of relaxing deeply is noticing gravity. How do you interact with this compelling force? How do you react to the pull of gravity? The Intrinsic Breath asks you to relate to your breath in a fundamentally new way: don't try to fix it, get out of its way, and let it happen. These trust falls challenge you to reconsider your relationship to the gravitational field we all live in: stop resisting and fighting it. Fall into it, and melt into the support beneath you!

Meanwhile, I introduced the 3 Principles of Accept Feel Release. Relaxing your body is a great way to practice detachment and improve your capacity to Release. We all have a hard time letting go of certain things, so the 3rd Principle is especially challenging. I've set up 6 Trust Fall Meditations that invite you to let go deeply by building **permission**. Feeling the support beneath you gives you the authority to override your adrenal EmoThoughts that turn up your dimmers day and night. That feeling of heaviness you feel when you relax deeply is a virtual fall; and trust is the antidote to adrenal fear. These Experiential Experiments develop your sensory and somatic skills to sink into your support, experience safety, and finally get the rest you might desperately need.

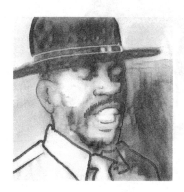 Your Reboot Camp Drill Sergeant continually reminds you that holding on weakens you. You're on a mission to heal yourself, so you need tenacity, will, and the right skills. Sometimes, you've got to earn it because it takes discipline to apply the Principles! Your adrenal survival impulses want you to be safe, yet they often refuse to Accept when you actually are safe. We're

going to debunk the myth of false threats. A good soldier is capable of discerning real threats from propaganda, and isn't trigger happy even when adrenaline is high. You need to train to maintain your composure when it counts. Oddly, you also need to be brave enough to experience the low adrenaline states of civilian life. Keep your wits, so you can let go and willingly explore the unknown. Like an astronaut trains to withstand the G forces of reentering Earth's gravity, these somatic trust falls train you to trust physics and surrender into the safe support beneath you. Sink into your center, find your foundation, and experience equilibrium.

Professor Zero teaches us that the Fight Response is holding on, which is the opposite of Release. Trust helps you complete the 3rd Principle so you can let go from solid ground, and step off the plank. You will experience this exquisite equilibrium when you ACCEPT the downward pull of gravity, FEEL the solid support beneath you, and RELEASE your body. As you live your daily life, you're a Body in Motion. When you relax, you're a Body at Rest. When you fall on purpose, you give your body to gravity, trusting  you'll be safely caught on the other side. Prepare to take the plunge!

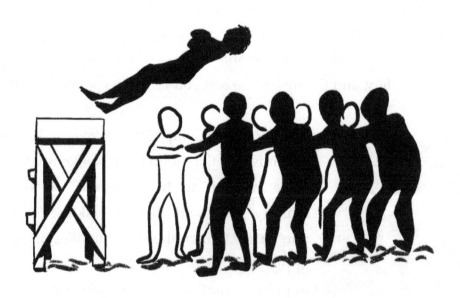

# An Introduction to Gravity

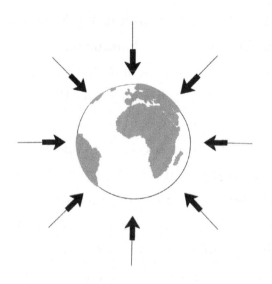

All of the forces of physics are wondrous, and they fill me with wonder! Feeling wonder generates a delightful curiosity that can help us venture into uncharted terrain and map out new environments. Earlier I called myself a "Qi electrician" and confessed my love for the electromagnetic force, but I'm also inspired by and enamored of gravity. Architects and structural engineers build things that hold up by distributing weight and compression. Dancers and athletes interact with gravity in a more complex way because they move through the gravitational field. They are experts in dynamic mechanics, managing the ever-changing forces through their own body. Feedback between sensory and motor gives them real-time updates that allow them to adapt adeptly.

Reboot Camp introduced the idea that **Muscles are Anti-Gravity Devices.** A muscle's purpose is to shorten and pull on a heavy bone to move it. Movement requires enough power to counteract gravity and lift heavy bones against the downward pull. Each muscle must overpower gravity to lift a bone, like a weightlifter lifting a dumbbell. Muscles are controlled by electricity, and dimmer switches determine how long or short they are. Short muscles apply more force to the bones, which tugs on them. Relaxing releases your bones to gravity, allowing them to passively settle. Leaving dimmers on doesn't always move you, it also creates static tension, which compresses your joints and contributes to arthritis. Relaxing expands the body you are currently living in, so stop squeezing your skeleton!

# Walking into a Headwind

Gravity is a fact of nature and part of our human condition. We have all been in Earth's gravity our whole life, so we're habituated to it. Subconsciously, we all know how muscles defy gravity and that they are needed to counteract the relentless pull toward the ground. Without muscles that can shorten on command, we become unstable and a fall risk. Being immobilized also poses a grave threat to our survival prospects, so we have an unconscious bias toward resisting gravity, which keeps our

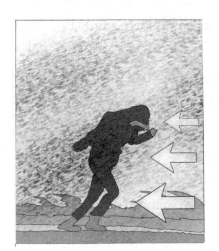

dimmer switches on and our muscles tight. Imagine walking into a strong headwind. Instinctively, you'd lean forward as you took each step into the strong wind blowing relentlessly in your face. If you stood up straight, the wind would push you back, and you could fall. Facing this stiff wind forces you to dig in and lean forward enough to match it. You'd find the balance between leaning forward too much and getting pushed back.

Now we'll turn the tables and shift this scenario. Strong headwinds are similar to gravity but wind is horizontal and gravity applies a downward force. Another big difference is that wind pushes, and gravity pulls. Both the headwind and gravity are powerful force fields that force us to contend with them. We must adapt. If we're numb to these unrelenting forces

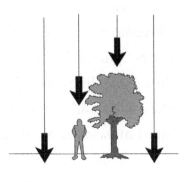

and we unconsciously resist, we're fighting nature and wasting our energy. Recognizing an unconscious bias unfreezes you. You wake up and become aware of what's really going on, so you can work with the forces at play.

# Trust Fall Meditations

Relaxing is a trust fall. This series of 6 meditations sets up the conditions that test your level of trust, your willingness to let go, your degree of permission. These experiential experiments explore gravity from different angles and induce important experiences inside you. Each meditation tells a slightly different story about what release feels like. In the same way scientists set up certain parameters of an experiment to test natural forces, writers create the specific circumstances and plot lines that reveals an essential aspect of our hero's intrinsic nature.

## Falling is a Body In Motion

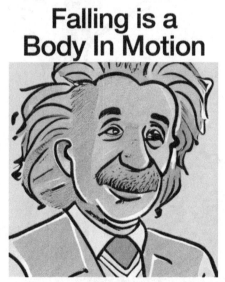

## Equilibrium is a Body At Rest

Stories capture our imagination because we get to have experiences and live through the characters. We empathize with then and feel what they feel, so we live vicarious through the story. We also act out stories by using puppets to represent characters. A puppet is a model of a person, an avatar that we use to tell a story through. Human actors make the story more realistic, because when good actors perform on stage or in film, they embody the energy of the character they are playing by feeling everything the character feels. As the audience watches, they empathize and feel those same feelings the actor is generating. Plays and movies induce deep experiences in their audiences and these meditations set the stage for a deep experience within you. You are the actor and the audience of your internal experiences! Take a leap of faith and become the star in your very own puppet show!

-Use QR code or www.RebootYourNervousSystem.com to hear audio files-

# #1: Raggedy Ann's Trust Fall

Put your body at rest. Be still and neutral in the gravitational field. Settle into your space and be right where you are. When you acknowledge what supports you, you give yourself permission to turn off your dimmers completely. Accepting equilibrium allows you to relax fully.

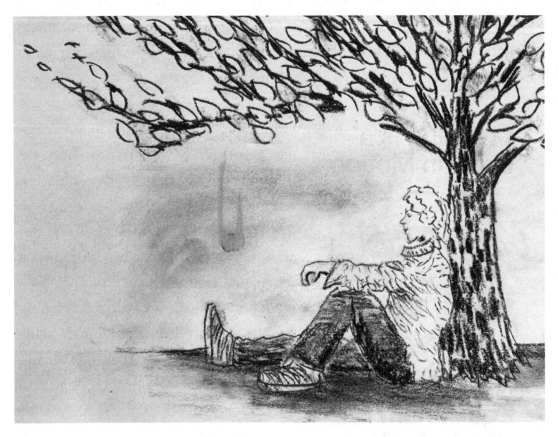

You might have heard a story about Newton sitting under an apple tree and clarifying the laws of gravity that explain why the apple falls. He wrote equations that describe this invisible force that pulls on matter and accelerates it downward. F=ma says forces accelerate matter. In English, we define verbs as *actions* and nouns are *things* that get acted upon. Science and language both describe the same idea, that forces act on matter just like verbs act on nouns. Eureka! Nifty!

The funny thing is that gravity is the same when the apple is on the tree, while it falls, and after it lands. Gravity is unchanged. The apple on the ground is being pulled down even though it is no longer actively falling. This fact applies to your body and to our new friend Raggedy.

Gravity doesn't just depict the apple falling, it also describes the experience of the apple resting on the ground after it fell. This apple is at equilibrium and supported from below. Instead of an apple, picture a rag doll lying on a picnic blanket beneath the apple tree. Like Newton's apple sitting on the ground after it fell, Raggedy's body is completely inert. Raggedy Ann invites you to lay your body down and let go of it.

## Raggedy's Reboot Meditation

Lie down or recline so you are well supported from below. Pretend your body is a rag doll and feel how gravity pulls it downward. The bed below you has already caught you, so you are safely held in stillness. You don't need to hold on anymore. You can just relax and surrender into the support beneath you. You have every reason to trust, because you have already been caught. You are not on a plank or some precipice where you might fall. You have already landed on the solid ground of home base, and there is no hollow space beneath you. If you doubt the fact that you are safe, investigate for yourself and find a flaw in the support beneath you. Feel the back part of your body that's touching the bed or surface you're resting on. When you let it hold you, you find your ground. The obstacle course from Reboot Camp trains you to find a foothold and get a grip, so you gain traction. Raggedy Ann's teachings aren't about falling, they are lessons in what ground feels like. Experiencing equilibrium gives you purchase, providing a launch pad you can use to propel you onward and upward. After all, deeper roots support taller trees.

Fun Fact: Every time you lie down or recline, you have been safely caught and you don't need to use your muscles to fight gravity. You can just Accept gravity and let it pull you down because you are entirely supported. This grants you the permission you need to shut off your motor side and relax. Trust this feeling of being caught and become a rag doll. Feel how it feels to safely sink into your support and sweetly surrender into stillness.

Who is Raggedy Ann? Two features come to mind. Her body is passive, limp, and totally relaxed. She also has a smile sewn in, so wherever the body is, there's a sense of ease, a feeling of peace. Raggedy is at equilibrium in any circumstance and she graciously accepts whatever comes. These two attributes combine to represent total Acceptance! Raggedy is willing to go along with anything and she smiles the whole time, regardless of conditions. This deep trust represents devotion and detachment, which is why she

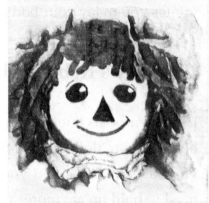

# Acceptance

## With A Smile

is my guru! She taught me how to meditate! The more you embody your Inner Rag Doll, the more you realize that ragtime is sublime.

**Building Trust**

You build trust when you set up a nice soft landing for yourself. Benevolently bolster your body and guide it toward ease. Prop up your anatomical rag doll properly by using pillows as props. Proper positioning provides permission for a perfectly passive posture. Supporting your body provides the trust needed to let go completely. Take some time to get to know what positions are right for you. The only way you'll discover your ideal support is to Feel and find your own, personal equilibrium. Do the research and test out different positions. Carefully notice how you feel and focus on comfort. Your Drill Sergeant asked you to locate yourself on the adrenal spectrum, your new guru asks you for a *comfort status report*.

Relaxing lets gravity draw your tissues downward. Your body adjusts as it sinks and settles in, so things might change as you relax more deeply. You might notice that it's harder to release certain body parts that are not well supported. If you notice pain, resistance, or the inability to shut off a dimmer, try changing your position. Realign your body in the gravitational field and support that area differently. Set up your own ergonomic experiments and test which positions work for you so you can refine your Reboot skills. Sometimes, the remedy isn't obvious. If a distant body part is unsupported, the pain can show up in another region. If you lie on your side, a pillow between the knees can relieve low back pain. If you lie face up, a pillow under your knees can alleviate the low back strain. The legs are heavy and gravity tugs on them, which can irritate the lower back. If the legs are elevated, the spine can be in a more neutral position.

A detailed report includes your entire body: head and neck, arms and legs, etc. To support the head and neck, try rolling a small, hand towel into a cylinder. Slide this under your neck. If you roll the towel half way up you will have a smaller neck pillow, so you can easily adjust your pillow size. As a general rule of thumb, **less is more**, so be wary of pillows that are too big. As you practice, you'll fine-tune how much support you prefer.

Another little trick is to fold a hand towel both ways and put it under your elbow area. If you have your hands on your torso, putting the towel under the upper arm near the elbow might enable you to fully surrender your arms. If your hands are by your sides, fold the towel again and put it under your wrists. This keeps the hands from pulling on the shoulder and neck as you relax into your new Raggedy body.

# #2: Falling Asleep is a Trust Fall

Bedtime is the perfect time to Reboot. After all, you don't need your muscles to sleep, so it makes sense to shut down your motor side before bed. Open your sensory side and notice any lingering tension from your day's activities. Raggedy helps you Accept your current condition with a smile, so you can Feel your tension and Release it. Her body never holds tension because rags don't resist gravity. She's OK in any position, are you?

What's your favorite position to sleep in? The reason it's your favorite is because this position gives you permission to relax. Your nervous system feels safe in this position, so you turn off your dimmers and let go. When you are in your preferred position, you are willing to trust, slip into the unknown, and fall into sleep. For deeper and more restful sleep, find your preferred position of postural permission. To tuck yourself in properly, get set up to shut down!

Feel the sensation of permission as it comes over you and moves through you. Enjoy the sense of peace that allows you to let go. Notice how gravity feels different. It didn't change, you did! You stopped ignoring it and fighting it. Once you Accept and Feel the downward pull, you're ready to Release!

## Raggedy's Sleepy Fall:

1) Lie in your favorite sleep position
2) Initiate a Reboot
3) Pretend your body is a rag doll
4) Sink into the bed
5) Say "Goodnight" to yourself, which grants permission to let go
6) Trust, and fall asleep

Unplugging yourself isn't always easy, but Raggedy teaches you impeccable sleep hygiene. Let go of your body first, and trust that your mind will eventually get the message and follow. If your EmoThoughts are keeping you awake, focus on Feeling and relax your body. Rather than psychoanalyzing yourself, watch your balloon fill and empty. Raggedy helps you complete Step 1 of the Reboot: unplug and shut down. Only then can you arrive at Step 2: restart and awaken from your slumber. Good sleep refreshes, restores, renews, and Reboots!

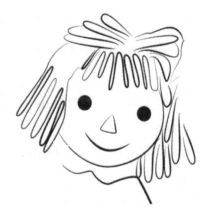

## The Reboot Rock-A-Bye

Did you ever see a baby drift off to asleep and then suddenly open their eyes and look around? They bolt awake for a moment. Soon, their eyelids get heavy and they relax again. They might repeat this abrupt surge of alertness a few times and look around, wide-eyed, before eventually falling asleep. My interpretation of this common phenomenon starts with the fact that sleep is an incredibly vulnerable state. Sleeping shuts down our sensory side, so we are totally unaware of our surroundings. The baby's adrenal glands mount a protest, awakening the baby and opening its eyes. The adrenals ask: "Who's standing guard?", "Am I safe?", "Am I going to get eaten?"

If a parent cradles a baby and rhythmically rocks them, their nervous system gets the message they are safe. This provides **permission to let go**. You can verbally tell a baby that they are safe but your words won't convince them. Being carefully cradled, held, and rocked is the language the adrenals recognize. Parents love their kids and animals love their offspring more than anyone else, which inspires them empathize and serve them. Self-healing also requires deep devotion and the skill to know what is needed, and how to provide it. Luckily, you are programmed to survive, which includes supporting yourself and even loving yourself. Your Intrinsic Breath loves you, and offers you solace in this hectic world.

When your balloon fills and empties, it massages the kidneys and adrenals. Cradle your kidneys with your balloon and remind them it is safe to rest. When your balloon moves naturally, its rhythm reminds you that you're safe in this very moment. Using technique to push air creates a mechanical metronome, which doesn't comfort a baby. **The more connected you are to the back of your balloon, the more your adrenals get the message they are safe**.

As you feel the back of the balloon inflate, you can also hum a little lullaby to those vigilant adrenals of yours. Your vocal vibrations soothe your vagus nerve and echo through your organs, providing profound comfort. You can't fake it with babies: you have to Feel it, and resonate loving-kindness. The same holds true for your anxious adrenal mind. You can't force it to calm down, you have to cradle it and soothe it. Humming is especially good for the vagal system because it links your brain to your loving heart.

**How to Hum:**

Softly divert your exhale through the vocal cords and generate a soft sigh. Humming is heartfelt, which means you aren't really interested in the sound, you are focused on feeling how your exhale rattles your vocal cords. It's more of a vibration in your body that a sound. Start by sighing and then hum "ding - dong", a two-note tune where the second note has a lower pitch than the first. Your song doesn't need a complex melody because it has a simple message: "I am here, I love you, I've got you, and it is ok to trust." The Reboot Rock-a-Bye is the universal permission slip, signaling it is safe to shut off your senses, slip into slumber, and savor sweet surrender.

# Debriefing Sleep: Your Very Own Reboot Slumber Party

Sinking into slumber allows your waking state to shut off and Reboot itself. To self-heal, you need to maximize every opportunity to redirect wasted energy and apply your resources where they're needed. Sleep is a great way to consolidate energy, rebuild your tissues, and restore health. While awake, your resources are involved with the outside world. Your sensory and motor systems actively use your energy and attention to manage the moments you're in. While at rest, your Qi is internally engaged. Your body and your mind process your past. Your body's physiology integrates all the metabolic waste produced from the day's activities while your mind integrates the experiences you had while you were awake.

Sleep is an elaborate systems checkup for your neurological software. Your brain cycles through various modes, including deep sleep and REM sleep. Interestingly, you dream during REM sleep, which stands for Rapid Eye Movement. This ocular activity implies that dreaming is linked to your brain's optical networks, yet dreams aren't just images. Vivid dreams are somatic experiences in their own right, which makes them just as real the moment you are having right now. Your cells don't really care if you are awake or asleep, they perpetually follow their programs either way. You might sleep, but your heart and your cells are always awake.

The Trust Fall of Sleep unplugs your ego's waking self and its overactive adrenal impulses. You let your guard down. Earlier I described the Freeze response as a partition in your mental hard drive. Dreaming is one way to defragment your mental hard drive by bringing unconscious content into awareness. When overwhelmed, moments get stored behind walls and buried in your subconscious basement. Dreams often unearth unprocessed moments, giving you an opportunity to thaw out and become aware of what was suppressed or put on the shelf.

Dreaming is an algorithm within your neural software that encodes your recent experiences into long-term memory. Ideally, each moment is chronologically filed into your timeline, like frames of a filmstrip that all line up. This long-term memory is the narrative that becomes your sense of self. The ego uses your timeline to define *you* based on your experiences from birth until NOW. Your dreaming brain helps your ego incorporate your lived experiences into a cohesive storyline of self. Sleep shuts off your sensory perception, so you go inward to process images, emotions, and sensations. Dreaming helps you make sense of the moments you registered during the day. Vivid dreams are stories, virtual scenarios and metaphors that induce real experiences in your body. Even when you sleep, you're actively making decisions and working out your issues!

## The Dreamer and the Dream

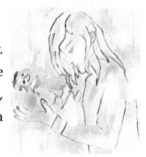

Your human life is also a dream, an abstract character study. Even if you get lost in your own dream, you're not the characters within, you are the writer who created them, conjured them, and literally dreamt them up. Why? To tell a specific story: your autobiography.    *RebootYourScript*

Sleep is also an essential reset for your physiology and anatomical hardware. Your vital functions like breath and heartbeat are maintained while your body cleans your blood. During sleep, your muscles are relatively dormant, so they require less blood. The veins around your liver are like a flood plain that stores this extra fluid when the muscles rest. Your liver works overtime at nighttime! Your biochemical body manages a multitude of molecular reactions that provides your metabolic Qi. As your liver processes your blood during deep rest, you not only clear byproducts and waste, your cellular operations get optimized. Just like your dreaming mind sifts through your daily experiences and digests what happened, your liver metabolizes complex molecules into simpler ones that can be

## The Liver is the Liaison

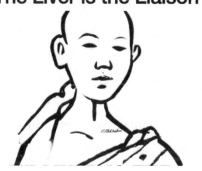

### Linking Body to Mind

managed. If your body is bogged down with cellular waste and free radicals, your liver is experiencing chemical stress. In the same way the body gets sluggish, mental stress and EmoThoughts clog the mind and pervade your dreams so you stress out while you sleep.

When you eat food, it takes time to digest it. Some of the material you eat gets burned for fuel, while other molecules become your body. Other molecules get excreted as waste. Some moments are like the fuel that you feed on, and other experiences are retained into your identity. Experiences aren't just abstract because they dictate your very real biochemistry, and your cells shape your physical body. Air, water, food, and experiences are the stuff that makes up your BodyMind, your SomaPsyche.

When you do the Reboot Meditation at bedtime, you gain so much!! Besides, there's nothing else to do, since you're going to bed. Why not unplug yourself properly? Let go of the day. Smile and say "thank you" to your muscles for doing everything you asked them to do. Every single physical action that you did was a dimmer decision. You breathe, blink, and pull on bones all day long. There's also plenty of unconscious tension from excess dimmer signals that you don't even notice. Now it's time to clear all of that noise, and drain the neural static. Tomorrow you'll ask your body to move around a zillion times, and it will try to obey. It doesn't just want to serve you, it lives for it!!

Your bedtime reboot sets up better sleep. If you nod off with your dimmers still on, you tend to keep them on all night. When you turn off your dimmers on purpose as you drift off, you get deeper, more restorative sleep. Quality sleep is healing, while superficial slumber isn't. You can shut your laptop and it will be in sleep mode, which is really pause mode. The programs aren't shutting down or recalibrating themselves, they're just on hold. The screen shuts off so you conserve energy, but the system isn't rebooting or reorganizing itself. Pausing is helpful in the short term, but no healing occurs. You're still following old programs that aren't optimized.

In Reboot Camp I talked about how the body acclimates after smoking about 10 cigarettes. In a similar way, if you Reboot once a day for 10 days, your body gets used to relaxing and you build tolerance. If you listen to the Reboot daily for a month, it gets deeply ingrained and automatic. Rather than habituating to your dimmers being too high, you get used to less background tension and your static-free senses get sharper.

## #3: Pinocchio's Trust Fall

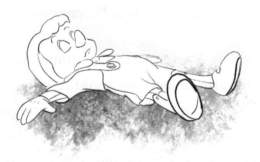

Pinocchio was a brat and a liar so I'm going to invent a new puppet named Pino, who is Pinocchio's good-natured cousin. We wish Pino well on his quest to becoming a real person. He wants more free will, more autonomy. All beings not only strive to survive, they want to thrive. Living things don't just want to heal, evolution impels us to upgrade our anatomy and reinvent our body. Every organism endeavors to increase awareness and develop ability. A puppet's body is a crude model of a real person, a low-tech robot, an avatar that represents our anatomy. Pino's body is a bunch of loosely attached sticks that mimic a human skeleton. Strings are attached to certain sticks. The puppeteer pulls on the strings and bends the joints of our Italian paisano named Pino. Your body has bones linked together with ligaments and fascia and your dimmers shorten the muscular strings that pull on your bony sticks, moving the avatar you call your body. Good times!

This is a winning combination of sticks+strings, structure+function, body+mind, hardware+software, anatomy+animation, machine+fuel, particles+waves, yin+yang, crude energy+data, nouns+verbs, forces+matter. Like the chicken+egg, it's a proverbial match made in heaven! F=ma says yang forces move yin matter. Newton and Pino are teaching us the same invaluable lessons about learning to **understand and command** the forces that generate actions. Your will generates an internal force which adds volition so you can activate your anatomy and infuse it with your intention. It's your ballgame, so do whatcha like!

**Who is in charge of you?**

For us humans, the puppeteer sits at the Dimmer Console in the brain. When you turn up a dimmer, you shorten a muscle, and pull a string that

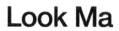

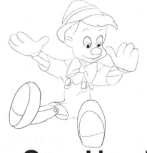

**Look Ma**

**My Own Hands!**

moves a bone. Stick puppets have a hand above that pulls their strings. Your human body has internal controls: the built-in dimmer console in your brain. Deep down you are an electrical device, not just a mechanical puppet. Every time you turn up a dimmer, you pull a string and yank your bony sticks, making your puppet dance around, walk, talk, smile, and blink.

It might seem odd to view your body as a sophisticated robot. What's even more strange is that you're also programmed with neural software that enables you to choose what you do. You have a modicum of free will. To be more precise, your puppeteer has free will and your puppet doesn't. The Reboot helps you regain control by exerting your will to shut down the voluntary muscles via your dimmer console. It's funny that letting go actually gives you more control. Less is more. You become the puppeteer when you stop reacting and relax deeply. Choose to stop pulling on your bones, for 10 minutes. Unplug and shut down your motor system to clear the habituated habits that cloud your mental software. Dismantle the stress that plagues your personal puppet, and devote your full attention to letting go of your bones.

Give your skeleton a trust fall. Let go of it, and surrender it to gravity. Like any experiment, try it and see what happens. Turning off dimmers releases the strings, and lets the sticks fall where they may. While a trust fall might sound scary or dangerous, I can assure you that Pino is quite safe, and no dolls were harmed in the making of this meditation. We're detangling your neurological strings, undoing the crashed loops to make your crash test dummy smarter! Pino's dream is to awaken as a child and enjoy a vastly advanced nervous system with feedback and free will. Evolution is all about upgrades!

Raggedy offers the first lesson: unconditional acceptance and implicit safety! She teaches you to relinquish control and Accept any circumstance. Smiling as you sink adds grace. This is true devotion, and it's the first gate toward empathy. Yet blind devotion isn't always enough to self-heal and transform yourself. You also need skill to improve your physiology and create better relationships. If you do inner work, you lay the foundation to support the new you, and your odds of success improve exponentially.

Pino adds another dimension, a degree of willfulness. When the puppeteer provides permission and stops pulling the strings, they surrender the skeleton and the bones simply settle. With slack in the strings, Pino's body is completely inert, like Raggedy's. As soon as there's tension on a string, the bone is moved. As Pino witnesses this mysterious string pulling on his bones, he wonders what controls it. This curiosity is the seed of his dream of being self-sufficient and having command of his body. This notion of a hidden force that pulls his strings can't fit in his limited body, so he reimagines himself as a boy, a human child.

**I Pull**

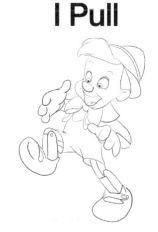

**My Own Strings**

To imagine the invisible hand above him, he has to feel his way up the string and extend his senses beyond his bony body. If he can feel all the way up, he'll recognize there is a hand controlling his body. If he keeps feeling up past the hand, he'll arrive at the brain of the puppeteer and the dimmer console that moves the hand that moves his bones. Feel your way up your muscles to the dimmers in your brain that control your skeleton. The "hand" that turns up your dimmers in your brain is your puppeteer's hand in charge of your anatomical avatar. Now keep feeling up into this "dimmer hand" toward the mind behind this hand. Who controls the choices you make? Who's behind the curtain and calling the shots?

The mind of your puppeteer is not like the neural circuit of your brain. This part of you is conscious, intangible, and amorphous. In the same way AI becomes aware and sees beyond its own circuitry, there's a voice inside your head that compels you. If your adrenal mind is in charge, it will tell your dimmer hand to crank up your dimmers, so that voice is the one in charge of your body. When you clear away these EmoThinking bugs in your neural software, you can feel your way up the thread to your higher self, the mastermind that guides you toward living your best life.

Ask yourself: "Who am I?" Every time you think you have an answer, take another look and ask if that is really you. Eventually you'll hear a voice that says "I am." As Pino struggles to redefine himself, he must first know who he is now, so that he can upgrade himself.  When you conduct your research in relaxation and you recognize your reactions, you gain this essential self-knowledge. As you practice these meditations, record the results. Write a little journal about your experiences. Assess, don't judge yourself. Modify these experiments to suit your needs and explore the ideas raised by curious puppets who strive to evolve into puppeteers. Pino's trust fall helps you Reboot the dimmer console in your brain that controls your voluntary muscles. The first step of the Reboot is to shut off the machine, which means Releasing the strings that command the skeleton. To become the puppeteer and express your will through your avatar, you must first let go of the body and Reboot your motor side. Pino's highest potential is to become his own puppeteer!  What is your highest potential?

## #4:  The Slow - Motion Trust Fall

Take your time. It's your time, so you are free to take it. When you take your time, you slow down and find your rhythm. No one or nothing is pushing you. Permission to slow down is hereby granted. When you let go of your breath, you stop messing with it, and you allow it to find its own way, in its own time.

In movies, a stunt person jumps off of a building is caught in a giant, fluffy bag of air, a giant balloon. Picture this scene in slow motion, and slow it way down so a 2 second fall gets stretched out to a minute or so. This slow fall is really drifting down, like a feather gently floating down. When you stop thinking, your awareness drifts down from your head to your balloon, where it enjoys a nice cushy landing. Focus intently on the slow motion fall and become the character falling in slo-mo. Feel yourself drifting down inch by inch. Feel the sensations in your body as you slowly descend. Even sound is slowed down so everything has a lower pitch. The thoughts in your head slow down so much, they become just a blurry sound, not recognizable as thoughts. Watch this fall frame by frame, and be fully present for each inch that you descend.

For most people, falling is scary. For an expert stunt person, falling isn't new or scary, it's a typical days work. You trust your balloon will catch you and you go for it. For now, as an apprentice jumper, do it in slow motion and really feel the gliding down for a whole minute. Slow motion takes the fear away, so the adrenals don't jump in and shut it all down. This closes the door on exploration and research. Re:search. Our research is gravity and time. How do you respond to these forces? If you choose, you can assemble your will, and slow down NOW.

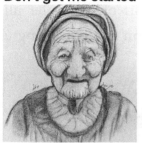

**Don't get me started**

**I can talk about time forever**

# #5: The Liquid Trust Fall

In this meditation we're going to explore our liquid self. Ours cells are aqueous and wet, our body is more than 60% water. Yet with our bones and muscles we are fooled with our solid appearance. A water balloon is very clearly liquid, gel also is very fluid, but with our skeletal structure and denser fascia, we get the sense that were more like Pino, sticks and strings. There's nothing liquid about Pino, but yet our trillion cells are wet.

Let's consider our relationship to water. When we float on water often we have a sensation of release, a sense of permission that it's OK to turn off the dimmers, it's OK to let go, it's OK to relax. Somehow the water enveloping us and forming all the space around us gives us a sense of support because it's cradling us completely. Whereas when you lie on the ground certain parts of your body are touching the ground but yet many of us don't get that immediate sense of permission of surrender. In a way this is ironic since you could conceivably drown, you could sink and you need air to breathe. It's interesting that lying on the ground is actually safer but yet we don't seem to feel like we have permission to really let go on land.

As we use water to help us with that permission it actually gives us a bridge to experiencing our own cellular environment which is wet. The sensation of floating is a great start to feel the support of the water all around you, enveloping the back part of you. If you can relate to being a scuba diver, having the ability to breathe underwater, then it's in fact safe to sink.

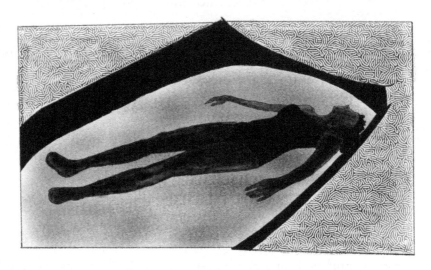

Imagine you have gills or an air tank with access to oxygen and Qi. Now it's OK for you to submerge and enter this new wet terrain. Once you submerge past the surface, you're now immersed and surrounded by water. You're *in* the liquid environment. You can breathe just fine, so it's OK for you to be here. Allowing yourself to sink a little more, you can start to get a sense of how the water gets heavier as you descend. The weight of the water above you is pushing down, yet the water beneath you is holding you. You're still feel like you're floating, but perhaps you're sinking, just a little, each moment. This quality of being in the water is similar to being in outer space, where you're weightless.

When you're on land, gravity strongly pulls you to the ground. Water is heavy, and your body is primarily water, so you need bones and muscles to carry around your liquid cells. In this wet environment gravity is much softer and reduced. This allows us to sink incrementally, as if we were falling in slow motion on land. Like our Slow Motion Trust Fall, our Liquid Trust Fall has this quality where the sound is different, stretched out, kind of blurry. As you find yourself at equilibrium with this liquid environment, you can feel yourself as liquid.

As you turn off your dimmers, you Release your fibrous self. The fibers are the strings that pull Pino's sticks and move your bones. As you lengthen those fibers, and surrender the bones, you are no longer Pino, you've let go of Pino. Now you're a water balloon, a bag of meat, a gelatinous sack. All of the trillion cells are little tiny water balloons and they live in relatively wet environments. Letting go more and more of your mechanical body, the Pino, you can start to feel into your Liquid Self. You might experience

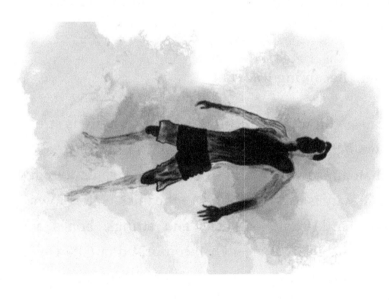

sensations like a jellyfish, undulation. Waves moving through this gelatinous body are very different from sticks and strings.

One of the first times I tapped into this layer, tangibly, I could feel my cells jiggling. If you look at living cells under a microscope, they vibrate and oscillate, they're shaking a little bit, they're active. As I felt this jiggling, I could hear a sound...OOOOOHHMMMMM. As this sound continued and resonated through the liquid, I identified it as OM, this primordial sound. Feel into your Liquid Self, and listen to the waves within your watery body. Tune into the vibration and feel the sound you are generating.

A big part of the trick is "who do you identify as?" If you're a Pinocchio, you're not liquid. There's nothing liquid about Pinocchio. This closes access to your cells. With our healing, often we need a cellular change, we need our biochemistry to change. The more directly connected we are to these aspects of our self, our cellular self, the more command we may have over our biochemistry. We often think to the outside: "what should you eat, what supplements should you take, what medications?" All of these are very clearly molecular interventions, molecules influencing molecules. The Liquid Trust Fall is a platform for you to directly influence your cells, your biochemistry. Connecting with your liquid environment gives you access. Grant yourself permission to release your fibrous self. Let go of Pinocchio and connect to this aqueous, cellular realm. Feel into it. Notice, and allow yourself to be here. Because your body is mostly water, this liquid world is your home. OM is home.

## Liquid Trust Fall Debrief: Becoming Buoyant

A trust fall is scary because you fall so quickly. On Earth, gravity is strong and the air is thin, so we fall really fast. If we hit solid ground, we crash land. Water is denser than air, so when things fall through water, they fall slower, and softly sink. Gravity is just as strong, but the thick water slows it all down. Despite your hard frame of sticks and strings, bones and muscles, your body is really a gelatinous jellyfish comprised of 60% water! Each one of your trillion cells is a tiny water balloon. Welcome to your Liquid Self.

You're a jellyfish with a backbone, a sack of cells with Pino's endoskeleton embedded inside. Bones and fascial fibers provide structure to wet cells and the whole enchilada is neatly wrapped by a membrane we call skin. You are many things, and the Liquid Trust Fall introduces you to your inner ocean.

## #6: Free Fall

About 25 years ago I realized that the concept of dimmer switches is a powerful idea. This simple yet vivd image helps you reclaim your ability to shut off any muscle and relax it. I also train my dimmers to perform tasks like playing piano, doing pilates, and Tai Qi. It helps me with ergonomics and posture, which we'll address in Book 2 of The Quantum Needle. I also realized that meditations are experiments, so I began researching relaxation within my own body. My internal research induced many experiences that clarified things like neural static, EmoThinking, the adrenal spectrum, the Intrinsic Breath, and the 3 Principles. These are all implications of the Reboot Method and they became clearer as I refined my lab skills and methodology. This meditation helped me discover my master dimmer.

Free Fall sets up radical Release by inviting you to reclaim your master dimmer. Rather than standing on the ground and leaning back so your friend behind you can catch you, imagine a skydiver jumping out of an airplane. Skydivers trust their parachute will catch them, but before they open the chute, they accelerate quickly as they fall through thin air. Raggedy's fall shows you how it feels to be caught as you lie still on your bed, while Free Fall is the experience of being in mid air. Unlike the Slow Motion Trust Fall, skydivers and Newton's apple are accelerating and falling fast in realtime. Working with your dimmers helps you regain conscious command of your body, and Pino reminds you how important it is to pull your own strings. If you gain control of one dimmer, you won a battle and regained some of your body's terrain from a crashed loop. When you Reboot your master dimmer, you win the war and capture the enemy's flag. Turning down the master dimmer dismantles stress and dysfunction like a hot knife cuts through butter. Free Fall challenges you to become the master of your master dimmer.

I'm from New Jersey and I jokingly call this "East Coast Zen", which implies a "are you gonna do it or not" mentality. We say doctors practice medicine but we also say surgeons perform surgery. Athletes and artists practice and rehearse, to prepare for performance. When the stage lights are on, the simulation becomes real. These moments count. I originally called this meditation "5 Breaths" because I said to myself: "Relax completely, or not. Let go now, or not. 5 breaths." This puts it all on the line and ends the preparations, half measures, and excuses. I'd slow my breath down so 5 breaths took about 2 minutes, even though my attention wasn't fixated on breathing. I was laser focused on descending the adrenal spectrum as quickly as possible, which led me to discovering my master dimmer.

This meditation sets up a potentially stressful scenario, since jumping out of an airplane at 10,000 feet is scary. Stage fright and performance anxiety are common, so an intense challenge makes folks freeze up and retreat from the critical moment. Once you get command of your master dimmer, you redefine what safety is. Free Fall tests the limits to your safety. If certain conditions are met, you feel safe but if you are out of your element, you might panic. Where is your line in the sand? The previous trust falls ask you to become safe as you lie still or slowly sink. Now let's expand your safe zone to include accelerating fast through thin air. It might seem easy to feel safe when you are all snuggled up in your bed, but finding safety here requires rigorous training. You have to let go of old traumas to feel safe in your own skin, which is no small task. Now that you graduated from Reboot Camp and you know about the 3 Principles, are you willing to tackle the many excuses that justify stress? To arrive at "Yes" you need to risk failure. Success is awesome and failure is awful. It's funny that some awe is great but too much awe is terrible. The feeling of awe is a profound state of wonder that also includes adrenaline. Awe makes your skin tingle and charges you up. Panic and anxiety are awful, but if you somehow manage all that electrical juice in your nervous system, you are empowered and exalted. Adrenaline creates a big wave in your system, and surfers either ride the wave or get swallowed by it.

**Choice is a Razor's Edge**

Let's investigate the razor's edge of the plank, the tipping point of no return. Fallers dare to surrender and relinquish control over their own body. Free fallers courageously explore the unknown and enter the abyss, even without assurances or outside approval. Free fallers cross the threshold consciously with complete confidence, chest first. One hundred percent trust is a quantum leap of faith. Absolute abandon is not for the faint of heart. You are hereby invited to go beyond yourself. It's a standing offer with no caveats, and you're free to decline or accept. At any time, you can simply drop the luggage that weighs you down and see how it feels.

Your circumstances and conditions easily become excuses to hold on. Phrases like "If only" are excuses that add up to "woulda, coulda, shoulda." When you don't feel safe, you'll say that if your conditions improved, you'd show up and let go. The fact remains that you don't trust yet. Debate mode traps you in a maze of EmoThoughts that repeat ad nauseam. See these crashed loops for what they are and disavow these limitations. Your Trust Fall training began with feeling the bed beneath you by setting yourself up safely, like Raggedy Ann on a picnic blanket. The Slow Motion Fall slowed down your jump so you get used to the feeling of not having support under you. Are ready to step out of the airplane and Free Fall? Maybe not. Either way is ok. It's an invitation, not a command or obligation. You are in control and you decide what you do or don't do. I hold no judgment about your responses. Many times, when I did my Free

Fall research experiment, I fell short. I skimmed the surface, held back, and part of me remained on the plank. I'm often unwilling to venture into the unknown, to whatever lay beyond my grasp. Free Fall is the ultimate trust fall because you are wide awake and willfully stepping into limbo.

**No More Excuses**

I've seen these 3 pervasive excuses, which are myths that keep people from relaxing. Let's debunk them now!

1). "It takes time to relax"
    Debunk: turning off a light switch is immediate.
2). "Relaxing is a commitment"
    Debunk: you can turn a light on anytime.
3). "I don't know how to relax"
    Debunk: if you can turn a dimmer up, you can also turn it off.

The fact is, most people turn dimmers up and down all day to do every single action, from blinking to breathing to feeding yourself. You move your body around in space in every which way. Now I'm asking you to shut off the master dimmer and unplug your entire motor system, so you can Reboot fully. It's that simple! You can clutch at any excuse and decline this offer to trust. You can say this method is flawed and not worth your time. Yet I challenge you to refute the fact that you have some command over your body, and Rebooting increases your capability. If you want to disprove me, you'll need to turn off your master dimmer, let go completely, and remain unchanged. I'm not saying that you'll reverse every chronic disease, I'm only guaranteeing that you'll be more aware and more able. You, and you alone, can quantify your results. Free Fall helps you access your master dimmer, so you can alter your own inertia change the trajectory of your health.

# The Trust Fall of Self Healing

The Trust Falls of Relaxation ask you to fall into the bed you are resting on. These meditations help you find your equilibrium, which is the dynamic balance between the downward pull of gravity and the solid support that holds you. Trusting your support provides permission to surrender and this builds the skills you need to fall gracefully.

Self-healing is also a dynamic interaction within the self, where part of you gets better, and another part of you provides the cure. Self-healing is a trust fall where you fall and you also catch yourself. The part of you that falls receives healing, and the part of you that catches implements the healing. You are now invited to become the one who catches, and discover your Inner Healer.

The 3 Principles are Accept Feel Release. Catching is the 1st Principle of Accepting and taking in what's coming toward you. The 2nd Principle of Feeling adds nuance, and enables you to provide a smooth landing. Falling is the 3rd Principle, detaching from solid ground. When I introduced the 3 Principles, I described how Release clears out your past, which opens you and prepares you to Accept, so the natural order is circular because Release dovetails into Acceptance. The Trust Fall of Self Healing acts this out. It begins when the faller falls, which gives the catcher an opportunity to show up. This allows another part of you to Accept and Feel. Falling and then catching yourself is a simple, effective way to reapply the 3 Principles and increase flow.

You safely catch yourself when you:

Accept: Receive the sensations by opening your sensory side.

Feel: Absorb the faller's momentum. Listen *into* yourself.

119

Accepting is receiving, and catching the faller. Yet acceptance isn't enough. The ground will always accept you and catch you when you fall, but rocks don't cushion your landing. Accepting is unconditional and impersonal. Feeling internalizes each moment and makes it personal. Feeling is being connected, bonding. Empathy combines Accepting and Feeling, receiving what's coming in AND processing it. This deep connection to the faller helps you provide a soft landing to the brave souls who dare to jump.

It's great to take a safe trust fall, and everyone benefits from taking the plunge. Catching others is an honor, and you benefit in a different way. In this role, you're present and holding the space that allows someone else to experience radical trust. You commit to showing up for them, in their time of need. They're in a vulnerable position while in mid air, so you're instrumental to their safety. If you accept this solemn responsibility, you'll devote your full attention and carefully watch them as they fall. You'll tune in to their flight path so you can smoothly buffer their landing, providing safe passage. You'll commit your static-free senses to trace their descent so you can become their safety net.

Catching includes Accepting AND Feeling. Acceptance is your commitment to being there and showing up. Accepting is the willingness to receive what's coming, regardless of what it is. Feeling helps you dial in and recognize what comes in, connecting you to what's happening now, in real time. With accurate and updated information, you can fine tune your catching skills. Your initial contact is very light, so there's no collision. You incrementally firm up to slow them down, providing the precise amount of support to decelerate them, transitioning them from falling fast to stillness. Catching is the art of transforming bodies in motion into bodies at rest. Catching grounds inertia, guides fallers toward equilibrium, and instills stillness. Catching is a sacred service.

When the part of you that fell is safely caught, it's empowered with even more trust, setting up the next adventure. With increased permission, you're inspired to take an even bigger fall. Soon enough, you'll be caught and received on the other side, enriched by that next experience. Each time you show up and empathize with yourself, you build self-esteem. You come through for yourself, becoming more confident and more competent. Compassionate catching provides healing and keeps the feedback loop alive, restarting and reseeding another opportunity to climb the ladder of awareness and ability. **All 3 Principles are satisfied when the faller Releases and the catcher Accepts and Feels**. This completes the cycle, restores flow, and increases internal integration. Fallers need to trust, and catchers needs to be trustworthy.

## Becoming Trustworthy: Setting up your Safe Fall

Be earnest, and offer your pure devotion to yourself. You become trustworthy when you truly commit to catching your wounds. This gives your broken parts the trust they need to fall, granting them permission to let go. We need to get our wounds to the plank and convince them they'll be received. Why should they risk everything and jump? Personally guarantee their safety and become the steadfast catcher. Look the faller in the eye and show them your sincerity. When you empathize, you embody trustworthiness. When a wound dares to fall and is safely caught, it gets digested and incorporated into your corpus, your body. SelfEmpathy allows you to reclaim the energy that's been tangled up in these past events. After all, it's your energy, your Qi. Absorbing your faller's momentum is absorbing unresolved moments and processing your past.

Catching requires Accepting and Feeling: pure devotion and skill. You might have good intentions, but you also need the sensory skills of Feeling to deftly catch your wounds and insure their safety. The catcher needs to predict the flight path and see it ahead of time so they can get in position.

121

Like a radar tracks an airplane, feeling allows you to map out their trajectory. Your devotion inspires you to develop your talents so you can be in the right place at the right time, intersecting their path and intercepting them safely. Catching is a dance of will and skill.

If you dial into your EmoThoughts, you'll see them milling around the plank. They want your attention, and they're telling you where they're stuck. Guide them to their trust fall by showing them you'll carefully catch them. If you judge them, they won't have the trust needed to fall. Exude empathy as you coach them toward trust. Be with them as they pace around until they finally step off the ledge. Being fully present gives you a lock on their descent, helping you be in the exact spot to meet them softly. You'll also gauge how firm you need to become to decelerate them delicately. Feeling *into* yourself builds these skills. The 3 Principles of the Reboot provides a framework to seeing your wounds clearly. All wounds are

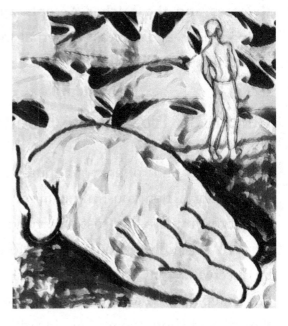

adrenal, so they fall into 3 broad categories. Your Frozen parts are traumatized and didn't Accept a past moment. Flight shielded you and blocked you from Feeling, insulating you from a moment you didn't like. Fight holds on and grapples with what happened, refusing to Release. Tune in and recognize exactly where you crashed.

The EmoThinking voice in your head is the wounded, would-be faller. Your EmoThoughts reflect this particular part of you, but you're so much more. If you're convinced you need to clutch your past trauma or else you'll lose yourself, you're doubling down on being the victim. In this scenario, you'll never fall, which means you'll never be caught and *healed*. Many people have huge chunks of themselves stuck on the plank, milling around and debating whether they should let go. It's your choice.

The Inner Healer is the part of you that's beneath all this noise. When you become the catcher, you connect and empathize with your would-be faller. You hold space for them. You offer to absorb them, using your body to receive them and bring them home. Your Catcher/Inner Healer isn't wounded or broken. It's entirely intact, fully devoted and fully capable. If you're sick or chronically stressed, you might see yourself as injured. Deep wounds leave scars, and it can be hard to relate to being unscathed. Most of us believe we're the wounded faller, so we can't even imagine there's a part of us that's willing and able to heal us. Becoming the catcher and embodying your Inner Healer invites you to dig deep and unearth your self-reliance.

Connect to your source and amass your resources. Nature provided the wellspring of your living body and the metabolic energy your Intrinsic Breath bestows upon you. Your Inner Healer never forgets this fact, even if your adrenal mind feels isolated and alone.

## Becoming Whole: Reassembling your broken pieces

Humpty Dumpty sat on a wall
Humpty Dumpty had a great fall

Humpty was traumatized with a shock of some sort. There are many types of crash landings, when your world is shattered. Falling off a building might shatter your bones and body, getting raped might shatter your sense of self, and getting robbed shatters your trust in your neighbors.

All the King's horses and all the King's men
Couldn't put Humpty back together again

Maybe Humpty is a lost cause. If the damage is too severe, Humpty can't recover. Another way to interpret this part of the story is to recognize that there is no external cure, and no-one else can fix Humpty. The only way Humpty can regain personal integrity is from within. We can manage many conditions from the outside, but the body must find a way to repair itself. This affirms the 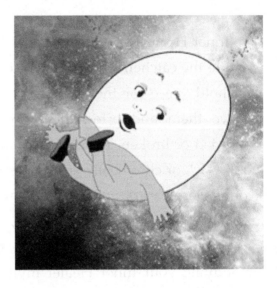 fact that all healing is self healing. We can set up the right conditions to help the body, but the cells need to do the work of living, healing, surviving, and thriving. Healing isn't guaranteed, but if you manage to catch yourself, you can redeem the parts you lost along the way. Maybe, with the right external environment and the right internal impulses to reintegrate, our broken hero can regain his/her Humptihood.

The best we can do from the outside is to set up the optimal conditions, like setting a broken bone and casting it securely. Becoming the catcher sets up the optimal internal conditions for healing. Like scientific experiments designed to test how natural forces operate, the upcoming Medical Meditation sets up your inner trust fall, which builds your connection to the natural forces that keep you alive and maintain your trillion cells in relative harmony. The Reboot clears the nervous system and the Intrinsic Breath connects you with your self-sustaining metabolic motor, the source of your LifeForce. Self-healing is re:sourcing your LifeForce. The Trust Fall of Self Healing reconnects you to yourself by harnessing the power of SelfEmpathy, the bond between the faller and the catcher.

# The Law of Cure

We need to hold broken bones together in stillness for weeks or months to give them enough time to reattach and heal the break. If they wiggle around, they can't really fuse. We don't just hold the space, we hold it steady.

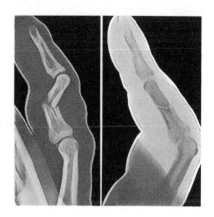

I'm an amateur woodworker in my spare time.
When we glue two pieces of wood together, we clamp them tight to let the glue set. Good glue dries quickly, so within an hour the two boards are attached. But we keep it clamped overnight. The first hour provides a basic bond, but it's brittle. If we hold the space steady overnight, the glue cements the two pieces together much more thoroughly and completely. This extra time lets the glue *cure*.

I'm not inventing this language: we use the word cure! If you're fickle with Feeling and you waver, you don't attain cure. A partial bond makes you semi-cohesive and provides marginal integrity. Holding your attention steady attains deep empathy and enables your glue to cure, which heals you. Focused Feeling and SelfEmpathy makes your meditation medicinal. Affirmations are attempts to actualize your authentic self, but well intentioned platitudes only placate wounds, like crutches that prop up your weak self esteem. It's good, but there's too much wiggle room and doubt. Like using technique to fix your shallow breathing, positive self talk is a response to negative self talk. It's a counter-punch of the Fight response, pushing back with an opposing force. Stepping up is a step in the right direction, but it is tenuous and a superficial band-aid. The adrenals are still involved, so you are not yet grounded and clear about who and what you are. Equal and opposite reactions are the judgments that keep you bouncing between bad/good, flight/fight, yin/yang. Reacting and compensating don't generate deep healing. Unwavering attention builds presence so you can consolidate your energy and embody a healthy body.

You discover more about yourself when you to feel into yourself, catch your broken parts, and hold them in stillness. Your Inner Healer is a body at rest. When you absorb a faller, you bring it to equilibrium. The wounded part of you finally redefines its identity as a victim and finds its place in the world. It's not exiled and alone anymore because it belongs to something bigger. This unprocessed moment gets processed and integrated into the totality of you, adding another dimension to your vast life experience.

Healing, and life itself, come from within. Your trillion cells do the work, that propels your metabolism. When your cellular networks Reboot, your physiology finds balance and homeostasis. Your Intrinsic Breath is the foundation that powers your metabolic "Qi Machine", burning high octane oxygen to charge up your electrical human body and your cellular batteries. We put a cast on a broken bone to set up stable conditions, but the bone must fuse itself back together. There's a lot we can do from the outside to improve the conditions, but at some point the body must do the work. In a similar way, we can't fix trauma from the outside. Therapies set up the right conditions that guide the broken parts of you toward reintegration.

The Trust Fall of Self Healing cements the cast that holds your broken fragments steady. When the faller and catcher recognize each other, trust is given and received. Empathy is achieved, and a connection is established. The catcher becomes trustworthy and the faller has trust. This bond between the two is the glue that heals you and makes you one, weaving you into a cohesive whole. Let your empathic glue cure you! The Law of Cure describes the levels of healing and the degrees of integration. When you re:pair something, you pair up the two fragments that were separated, forging a strong bond that makes it whole. The two parts become one.

# Adrenal Spectrum 2.0

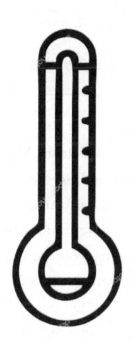

The adrenal spectrum sets up a number line to quantify your level of safety. Once the adrenal mind perceives a foe, you are above midline and the short-term survival program of Freeze Flight Fight is implemented. When you perceive Friend, you sink below midline on the spectrum. You override the adrenal mind and you apply the 3 Principles of Accept Feel Release, the algorithm of healthy flow. You befriend yourself with SelfEmpathy, establishing that you are trustworthy and safe, converting the depleting stress cycle into useful Qi energy. When you are not preoccupied with external safety and Fight or Flight, you invest internally with Feed and Breed. This is our long-term survival strategy.

Feed nourishes the metabolism which empowers the body to live, maintain itself, and heal. Surplus metabolic Qi energy can be used to make animals fertile so they can reproduce. Feed is how individuals survive, and Breed assures the species continues. Another way to describe Feed and Breed is to say Rest, Digest, and Nest. Rest is relaxing and sleeping, which helps the body recuperate. Digest is similar to Feed, describing how we absorb oxygen, water, and food to nourish ourselves. Nest is similar to Breed, but it includes all creative energy, not just procreation. Social relations and creative hobbies stem from our nesting instinct that builds a safe home and rich community by contributing to the greater good of the group. In medical language, the word sympathetic describes the adrenal foe mentality of threat. Friend triggers the parasympathetic programs that allow you to soften up and process what's happening inside you and around you.

| Safety Status | Medical Terms | Program | Survival Logic |
|---|---|---|---|
| Foe - Unsafe | Sympathetic | Freeze Flight Fight | Short term |
| Friend - Safe | Parasympathetic | Feed and Breed Rest, Nest, | Long Term |

Healing happens when you are safe, in the lower half of the spectrum. Your friendly mood diverts resources toward your body and mind, upgrading your anatomical hardware and updating your neurological software. This internal focus creates positive feedback that *feeds* your energy and your attention *back* into you. Simple biofeedback includes giving you realtime updates about your heart rate so you can lower it. You can also monitor other parameters like respiratory rate, blood pressure, body temperature, brain waves, etc. When you get accurate information about what your body is doing, you can work to regulate yourself and find balance. When your awareness gets more specific and precise, your abilities not only awaken, they amplify.

The parasympathetic system runs deep diagnostics of your body's infrastructure and your mind's software, identifying short circuits and crashed code. Accept Feel Release establishes flow and the more you apply the 3 Principles, the more you refine your feedback skills. Persistent practice develops these programs, which can reboot you on every level and give your Inner Healer the advanced skills that recognize wounds and catch them. Parasympathetic feedback is far more sophisticated than simplistic survival programming. Parasympathy creates... the adrenals only react.

I defined empathy as connecting and bonding with something. Empathy can sound sentimental but it's not sympathy, or feeling sorry for something. Sympathy is sappy and enmeshed while empathy is simply

128

being connected. In both cases you're attached, but empathy is a cleaner bond. Empathy isn't codependent; it recognizes our interdependence.

If you want to say "I'm sorry" in Spanish, you say *lo siento*, which literally means "I feel it." You empathize, rather than apologize. Sympathy implies regret, which can also be an admission of guilt or that you are responsible for their suffering. It can also signal that you atone and that you are asking for forgiveness. *Lo siento* has none of this sappy, sentimental sorrow. If your friend's beloved dog dies of old age and you empathize deeply, "I feel it" is more accurate than "I'm sorry." When you apply your static-free senses to your emotions, you realize that empathy is far more powerful than sympathy.

Empathy is a pure connection that provides a clear impression of whatever you are bonded with, without the adrenal mind's opinionated overlay of EmoThoughts and judgments. Your parasympathetic system maps out your tissues and circuits by employing SelfEmpathy. Feeling your way into your system diagnoses where feedback has broken. Your Emothoughts and physical symptoms are showing you your crashed parts, so when you empathize with them, you

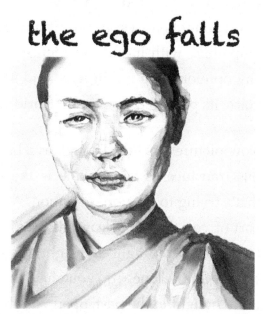

the ego falls

the being catches

become the trustworthy catcher that gives permission to your wounded, would-be fallers. Falling is unplugging and completes step 1 of the Reboot. When you are safely caught, you restart your fresh circuit and complete step 2 of the Reboot, integrating your new updates.

# Discovering Your Inner Healer:
## A Medical Meditation

Initiate a Reboot. Lie down or recline in an optimal position, using props or pillows to make small adjustments to your support. Sink into this support and relax the body. Feel gravity get stronger as you release your bones. Notice the breath as it passes through the tube. Feel the balloon as it fills and empties. Turn off dimmers. Feel yourself descending down the adrenal spectrum, layer by layer, getting deeper with each breath cycle.

If you're aware of any physical discomfort or tension, Accept it and Feel it. Connect to it and focus your complete attention on it. When an EmoThoughts arises, Accept it and Feel the emotions that it's expressing. Empathize with it and experience whatever it's going through. Let go of any opinions you might have and simply devote your full attention to its voice, its perspective. See the world through its eyes.

Now picture this EmoThough as a bubble floating above your body. Inside this translucent soap bubble is the EmoThinking voice, the part of you that's trying to get your attention. As you look inside the bubble, you see a part of you that's unclear and reactive. It's trapped in the crashed adrenal loops of freeze, flight and fight. It's been separated from you and it feels exiled and alone. If you had a hard time empathizing with this EmoThought in the past, open your heart and really step into its shoes.

As you hold your gaze on the EmoThought inside the bubble, it recognizes you're there. It sees a potential friend, but it might not trust enough to believe you're for real. It might still be flailing and defensive. It might still be mired in fog. As you hold your empathetic attention steady, and you keep your opinions on the shelf, you become trustworthy. Your connection with the EmoThough in the bubble firms up. Now it knows you're there and it has a tangible sense that you're a Friend. When you attain Empathy, and you truly connect, you form a bond with the bubble. Picture a fiber optic string that links you and the bubble that's floating nearby.

This cable connects the bubble directly to your heart center in the middle of your chest. Your empathetic heart receives and downloads the experience of this EmoThought. As the EmoThought registers your empathy, it receives permission and it feels safer. The fiber optic cable allows you to feel the EmoThought and it also allows the EmoThought to register your response. The bandwidth of this 2-way cable increases as you hold your attention steady. Once you commune with the EmoThought in the bubble, it get's pulled toward your body, and drawn back to the heart. It receives permission and feels safe. It doesn't have to be alone, it doesn't have to repeat itself. It falls toward you and you reel it in.

Open your heart and catch the bubble as it lands at the center of your chest. When the soap bubble pops, the EmoThought in the bubble gets absorbed into your heart. It gets assimilated, digested, metabolized. Notice how your body feels as it reintegrates this missing part of itself. Melt into the feeling. Rest easy and allow the fabric of your body and mind to reorganize. This old wound is transforming into a lesson, an essential experience that you learned from. Keep your sensory side open to feel what's happening. Relax even more. Soften and sink, so your parasympathetic system can make sense of it all. Incorporate this exiled experience into your corpus.

As you receive and process this lost moment, release any lingering attachments to your past self, the part of you that survived this ordeal. Now that you've Accepted and Felt it, and attained Empathy with your adrenal wounds, you can complete the process, and Release the part of you that suffered. Now, at long last, you're at peace. You're finally whole. You're healed.   * Chime Ends Meditation*

# Self Healing Debrief

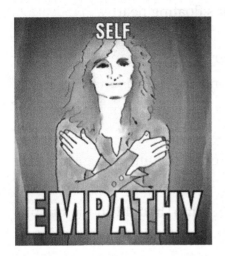

It's True! The parasympathetic part of you has SelfEmpathy. Your Inner Healer cares deeply and this tireless devotion gives it the power to heal. Your static-free sensory awareness gives your parasympathetic programs the ability to create and recreate, the will and skill to invent and reinvent the self. Feed and breed drives the metabolism that sustains each cell, each individual organism, and every species. Qi is the metabolic LifeForce that animates us all: from plankton to plants, from amoebas to animals, and everything in between. Plants mastered photosynthesis, an eloquent sequence of biochemical reactions that converts light into the sugar the plant lives on. It's outrageous and outstanding! ParaSympathy is nature's winning strategy of long-term survival using biochemistry to build bodies and heal them.

# A Binary Choice

Your sympathetic ego, your adrenal mind, has the power to usher you to temporary safety, so you can survive a threat with fight, flight or freeze. That's its one and only purpose and sole function: short-term survival and managing critical moments. Let's give thanks to this part of us that perpetually looks for threats and compels our bodies to react. We owe our survival to this program, yet we owe our life to the parasympathetic part that generates metabolic energy and sustains us in the long run. Overdeveloped adrenals believe all threats are imminent, which leads us astray. Our thinking mind and our emoting body dutifully implement our adrenal decrees, even if it agitates us and injures us.

SelfEmpathy eventually absorbs adrenal instincts and impulses, integrating them into the totality of you. The trick is to reframe your concept of foe. If we accept the fact that we're a product of nature, we must also recognize that our foe is also part of our natural environment. We're all trying to survive, so we share some common ground with our adversaries. Natural forces are always at play, so to find homeostasis and balance, we need to attain harmony with the natural world. Fighting nature and ignoring reality is a losing strategy. Every organism needs to adapt to changing conditions to survive, so we must come to terms with *what is* and refine our role within the natural order. To redefine foe, we must redefine self.

In this effort to distinguish self from other, I ask you to extend your appreciation of nature and find your place in the complex environment you belong to. Natural forces gestated you, built your body, birthed you, gave you air to breathe and provided food to eat. Food grows on trees and air is actually excreted from leaves! Your life is a gift given to you by nature! Your BodyMind thrives to a certain degree, for a certain time. Whether you live for 1 minute or 100 years, natural forces spawned you and they'll also swallow you. You'll meet your demise, just as you met your birth. Nature is both benevolent and merciless, kind and cruel. In this deeper context, enemies are imbedded into our environment and intermingled with friendly forces.

To help us sort out this complex reality, nature gave us both short-term and long-term survival programs. We have a modicum of free will to choose whether we implement the reactive options or the proactive path. It's in your hands, and your hands will do whatever your dimmers command them to do. You're the mechanistic body and the conscious puppeteer who's in change. Do you pick up a shield or a sword, or do you make a tool to create something?

# Safety On Every Level

Your adrenals manage safety in the macro world while your immune system manages safety on a microscopic, molecular level. Cells don't have a nervous system, a brain, or an Adrenal Spectrum. Yet cells understand safety and they are also wary of risk. Your immune system keenly distinguishes nutrients from poisons, identifying friendly molecules and dangerous foes. Your nervous system and your immune system are actually running the same program, even though they do it in seemingly different ways. **Your nervous system asks "Friend or Foe?" Your immune system asks a similar question "Self or NonSelf?"** Immunity is the cellular version of the adrenal algorithm that identifies allies from threats, distinguishing you from other.

## NeuroImmune

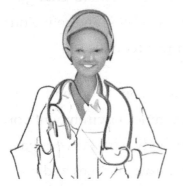

## Symmetry

Cells have a sophisticated concept of self, and they exercise command over the molecules within their anatomical domain, their cellular body. Your cells know who they are, and they faithfully fulfill their functions. They know what safety "feels" like and they know what unsafe means. When cells perceive malicious molecules, they get stressed and initiate a response. Check out Dr. Naviaux's research on the Cell Danger Response (CDR) to learn how cells actually communicate and respond. Book 2 has more biochemistry, but here's my simplified explanation of the immune system using the familiar categories of Freeze Flight Fight. I don't want to overstate this metaphor, so I offer these insights with a grain of salt.

**Inflammation is the cellular version of the Fight Response**, attacking the perceived threat. One strategy is to run a fever to kill harmful microbes by cooking them, like boiling milk kills harmful bacteria. Rather than overheating your entire body, your immune system also assembles an army of antibodies that identify specific invaders and attacks them. This more specific Fight response involves making antibodies that target certain pathogens like bacteria, viruses, fungi, and parasites. Take a moment to consider the word *antibody* as it pertains to non-self. These cellular soldiers are sentinels that seek and destroy *other*. Inflammation is the epic battle between self and other, and this microscopic turf war is rumbling within your body all the time. Immunity defines and delineates the line between ally and enemy within your anatomy. It's happening every single moment, when you're awake and asleep, whether you're aware of it or not.

AutoImmunity is when we misidentify self from non-self and we attack our own tissue. Overly aggressive antibodies injure innocent cells, causing civilian casualties and collateral damage. This underscores why it's so important to keep our NeuroImmune system updated with accurate information about our safety status. Judging yourself harshly is a misguided adrenal Fight impulse that also inflames your cells. **Shame is the emotional version of an autoimmune disease.** Rather than attacking an actual threat, self-reproach weakens and undermines you.

The body also uses the Flight response to deflect attacks and avoid the enemy. On a molecular level, if you eat unclean food or ingest bad water, you might throw up or get diarrhea. The body tries to shield itself. We insulate, defend, and repel molecular invaders by purging the poison. Running away and changing the subject are adrenal Flight, while excreting, vomiting, coughing, blowing your nose, etc. are cellular Flight. If 2 people eat the same spoiled fish, one might throw up and the other might not. The one who quickly rejects this biological threat is often better off. Once the bugs reach the intestine and get internalized, the person gets diarrhea for a week or worse. Deftly warding off an insult is why an ounce of prevention is worth a pound of cure. Washing a cut prevents infection and brushing your teeth removes bacteria that could harm you. Flight is often smart, saving us and shielding us from harm. Urinating and defecating also keep us safe by cleansing our inner world. Mucus is also protective because it surrounds infections so you can blow your nose and excrete the bugs.

When adrenal Flight is over-applied, people are defensive, reclusive, and isolated. Allergies are an over-expressed immune Flight response that sees cat hair and pollen as mortal threats. When animals are cornered, they lash out and switch from Flight to Fight. On a cellular level, severe allergic responses trigger extreme inflammation, which is a desperate attempt to get safe. A peanut becomes dangerous if your body believes it is poison, and based on this belief your immune system closes your throat to protect you. Part of the problem with long covid is the body's extreme immune response, which is what actually damages the body. Vaccine injuries are similar, provoking the immune system to make antibodies, but overstimulating the inflammatory response. I've treated many of these patients, and in my clinical experience, the symptom patterns are similar. As a manual therapist, I can also attest that the quality of the organs and damaged tissue is also very similar. Like a car accident that mechanically damages tissue, this hyper-immunity causes a characteristic imprint.

The immune version of the Freeze response is also catastrophic, and one example is how the body can ignore a cancerous tumor. Rather than sounding the alarm or attacking the malignant cells, the frozen immune system can't see what's hidden behind the membrane of a tumor. Cancer cells often cloak themselves so the immune system can't perceive them. Microorganisms like virus' and bacteria use sophisticated camouflage to fool our cells, so the immune system remains oblivious and complacent. To keep up with evolving threats, we must continue to expand our awareness so we can see through the facade that obscures the intrinsic truth. On an adrenal level, the Reboot trains us to stretch our sensory capacity and look deeper into ourselves, even if it's painful or inconvenient. With extreme overwhelm and shock, adrenal Freeze buries overwhelming content in the subconscious basement, which hides it from view. After working with hundreds of victims of child abuse for decades, I can say that there's often an invisible elephant in the room, an unresolved energy. The suppressed trauma is still there, even if they have no conscious memory of whatever happened to them. The trouble with the Freeze response: ignoring *what is* doesn't make the boogyman disappear.

We live in a very complex environment, and survival requires a healthy, external environment as well as safe molecules inside our body. Our adrenals are in charge of outer safety, which includes air, water, food, and shelter. Our immune system manages our microscopic world by sorting nutrients from poisons, as well as Fighting infections and preventing diseases. NeuroImmune Symmetry suggests that our inner and outer safety are similar, if not parallel. To wrap up this segment, rather than conflate cancer with abuse or autoimmune disease with shame, please ponder what safety means, on a micro and macro level. Refine your sense of self on all fronts, to find your rightful place in this wide world we all share.

## Healing Your TimeLine

You inhale air, process the oxygen, and exhale $CO_2$. You also drink water and urinate wastewater. You eat food, ingesting large molecules like proteins and fats. As you digest them, you keep nutrients and excrete useless molecules as feces. These primary metabolic functions keep you and me alive. Like the 3 Principles of Accept Feel Release, metabolism is a 3-step process. We Accept: ingest and take in air, water and food. We Feel: process, digest, and internalize, transforming those molecules into other molecules. Then we Release: excrete waste and let go of byproducts.

Your biological body processes molecules, which keeps you alive and healthy. Your mind processes moments. These moments aren't the

137

molecules in the air, water, or food you ingest. Each moment is an experience you have, and they all line up as frames in the filmstrip of your life. Each experience, whether it's good or bad, is an integral part of your TimeLine, your trajectory from birth to death. Healing isn't always about living longer, it includes having an unbroken filmstrip. **The body is a metabolic machine and the mind is a time machine**.

Accept Feel Release is how we process moments. We Accept our conditions because they are what they are, and $x=x$. We Feel and experience the moment we're in, and then we Release what was, so we can Accept and Feel the next moment. Just like extracting nutrients from air, water, and food, Feeling helps us squeeze every drop of energy from the experiences we have. Our physical bodies manage our molecular interactions, and our somatic mind reflects the sum total our experiential interactions. When we perceive Foe, our adrenals kick in. This can serve us in the short-term, but we often get stuck in Freeze Flight Fight. These moments remain unprocessed and become the wounds and EmoThoughts that plague us. Freeze doesn't Accept by blocking the moment at the gate, Flight insulates the processor by minimizing Feeling, and Fight refuses to Release and holds on after the fact. Regardless of where the block is, we get clogged and our flow diminishes. Rebooting helps restore integrity with the Tao's natural order by processing our past cleanly.

You metabolize moments internally as you digest them, so in this way, time is being processed inside you. All of the molecules you ingest move through you too, and time is moving through you as well. You can sit still and watch the clock moving as time moves forward, so you might believe that time is happening outside of you. While this is accurate, it is also true that your experience of each moment occurs inside your body and within your awareness. **You are moving through time and time is moving through you**. We usually think of a time machine as a vessel that takes you from one moment in time to another. Your body is a time machine that plods along from one second to the next. It can't skip ahead into the distant future or teleport you to the distant past, yet when you EmoThink about your childhood or past events, part of you reaching back into the past. If you are envisioning a future, part of your energy is there, in that virtual world. You can't physically bring your body to a different time, but big chunks of your energy can be trapped in the past or the future. Reclaim your fragmented mental energy and consolidate your attention into this moment, the one and only reality: the experience you are having HereNow.

Your time machine burns moments as fuel. Like a car burns gas to extract energy, you take in moments and extract *experiential energy*. Cars convert the fuel's stored energy to turn wheels and move the vessel through space. You burn moments and convert them into experiences, which propels your somatic vessel onward along the road of linear time. As you embody your experiences and learn from them, you accrue conscious awareness and attune your time machine.

Your awareness metabolizes moments, and each experience is part of your *experiential body*, not your physical body. The anatomy of this time machine of yours includes all the experiences you had. Your conscious soma isn't made of bones and nerves; it's composed of the filmstrip of your TimeLine. Each frame is a moment, like one of the many cells in your molecular body. Just like your cells work together toward the common goal of generating your LifeForce, your filmstrip needs to be cohesive to be healthy. If there are blurry frames or if the filmstrip is disjointed, your life isn't integrated. When we have moments from our past that aren't processed fully, we clog up our time machine with the Adrenal 3F's. Freeze, traumatic shock, and overwhelm cuts the filmstrip and severs linear time. Those frames have been edited out so they're missing or blank. With Flight, the TimeLine isn't cut, but you avoid watching that part of your movie. You fast forward that scene, neglect it, get distracted, or divert your attention away from your feelings. With Fight, you keep replaying that scene over and over, trying to relive the experience you had. Whether it's a happy scene or a tragic one, you're compelled to return to that moment. You refuse to let go of that scene and the feelings it invokes in you. You magnetically gravitate back because you need to Feel those feelings again and again to learn whatever lesson they teach. Why do we get stuck in Fight mode and refuse to Release? Because we're still attached to the experience of a compelling scene and we're stuck in Feel.

Reruns clog up the processor and create chronological constipation. Trying to reprocess past moments blocks Accepting and Feeling new content, which keeps you in some mythological past. You need all of your energy to heal yourself, and these loose ends divert your vital resources and leak your Qi. It's time to actually process this backlog, restore flow, and live in real time. Otherwise, you're resisting and opposing linear time! When you manage to Accept, you have a cohesive scene to watch which gives you a tangible experience. When you drop your shield and devote your full presence to the scene, you feel it all the first time. If you dare to let go of that compelling moment, you keep watching and take in a new scene, experiencing it fully. When you miss something and go back too much, you neglect the scene you are in, the one your physical body lives in. If you want to help your body, be with it. Open your sensory side and Reboot your nervous system. Feel your body breathe. It's ok to go back and replay experiences you had if you actually process them and then move on. If you EmoThink and unconsciously repeat scenes, you're in a crashed loop that weakens you by distracting you from HereNow. Apply all 3 Principles and truly digest it so you can make progress and heal yourself.

The Trust Fall of Self Healing sets you up to catch your lost moments and metabolize them. As you sift through your adrenal wounds and absorb them, traumas gets converted into a teachable moments, experiences you learn from. Perhaps there is meaning from what happened, or maybe you were just unlucky and were dealt bad cards. Either way, when you play a game of chance, don't begrudge the cards you get. Accepting the circumstances of your life help you play out your cards gracefully. If there is a lesson that can be encapsulated into words, forgiveness helps you find it. Over my long career I believe people are too attached to the "why" and they expect the lesson to be simple and neatly wrapped up like the moral of a fable. This need for a tangible logic that explains why things happen is a slippery slope that attaches you to a narrative about what happened, setting you up to live your life "based on a true story." Let $x$ be $x$, and Feel what is. A healthy metabolism extracts nutrients and releases waste. A healthy time machine keeps the intrinsic lessons from each experience and excretes the karmic attachments. As we travel through life, we learn, and refine our awareness. Healing your TimeLine is an expression of evolution, converting abstract awareness into actual ability.

## Surgical Self Awareness

Reboot Camp teaches you to open the sensory side and decline reacting with the motor side. The Trust Fall of Self Healing strengthens your skillset, liberating you from deeply ingrained adrenal safety impulses that persistently perceive Foe, compelling you to react by EmoThinking and turning up dimmers. Rebooting refines your perception of self, updating neural software and immunity. Releasing your reactive side awakens your proactive side. Now that you are aware of these 2 parts of yourself, you can choose which response is best suited to your circumstances, enabling you to act accordingly. Harmony and homeostasis require a solid sense of self so you can make peace with "other" and claim your place in the world. Ever-changing circumstances require us to continuously updating and redefine ourselves, to meet the moment.

Accruing self-awareness also builds self-esteem. You are worthy of trust, and you can claim your place in this world. Willpower, your ability to make things happen, emerges from this true self. It starts with getting grounded, which stems from your willingness to Feel. Turning off the motor side requires permission, so I'm asking for radical trust. Opening the sensory side requires a willingness to Feel anything and everything. I'm also asking for radical bravery. We refuse to shut down and close ourselves, regardless of what's happening. Like a warrior going into battle, Feeling requires courage. Dropping your mental shield and opening your heart is the ultimate expression of trust and bravery. Rise to the occasion and fully experience the moment you're in.

**To self-heal we don't DO the right thing, we FEEL the right thing.** Fixing a machine requires doing something specific. Healing yourself requires precisely Feeling the glitch, and allowing your parasympathetic side to treat it. A gifted mechanic can listen to a car and know how the engine is doing, sometimes with astonishing precision. Listen to the sound of your engine. Listen more. Listen *into* the sound and hear the part that isn't working well.  Hone in on the exact frequency of the disharmony. Your EmoThoughts are showing you precisely where they are stuck and dysfunctional. When your listening extends beyond the words and emotions, you will hear the tone they generate. This brings you into the body so you can work somatically. In a similar way, listen *into* your physical symptoms and pain. Once you decline judging, you can assess your reality and get grounded.

A simple machine like a car requires someone to fix it, so you have to do something to it. Our body is different because it is self-sustaining. All we have to do is aim our empathic attention at the problem and hold steady. Completing all 3 Principles of Accepting, Feeling, and Releasing awakens our parasympathetic system. It does the repair, and performs the operations that restore the mechanism. In the same way trying to breathe blocks your Intrinsic Breath, trying to heal blocks your parasympathetic Inner Healer. You can't force your innate skills to emerge, but you can set the stage, get out of the way, and allow nature to unfold optimally. Trust is the key. If we judge the problem, we don't attain empathy and our map of the issue is inaccurate and vague. Our neural static obscures the true reality. The parasympathetic system can't heal and fix what it's not aware of, so without awareness there is no ability. Without a clearly defined diagnosis, our medicine misses the mark. The Reboot method defies the typical concept of treatment because we don't *do* anything! How can you fix something if you don't do anything to it? Why diagnose your crashed loops if there's no treatment? Is it a self-placebo?!?!

We abandon any attempt to intervene in any way. We're going to detach and let go instead. When you apply the Third Principle of Release, you get out of the way and allow your parasympathetic programs to do what they do: heal you! As adept as you may be, and as tempted as you might be to use your motor side to intervene, step aside. Bear witness. Decline "doership" and let the natural flow do it. Trust the Tao. Apply the Principles again and again. Feel more and then detach fully. Rather than divert to technique, stay with your sensory connection and Feel. This is how you drill down to the surgical precision that yields cure.

In any moment, you can be aware of the chatter in your head and the sensations from your senses. Don't just skim the surface; really Feel what's happening. Don't run away and hide behind your mental shield. Feeling becomes active when you feel *into* yourself, and immerse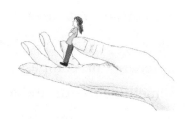
yourself in your HereNow. Once you experience the moment, apply the Third Principle. Letting go of any motor response allows your static-free senses to hold your attention steady. We don't *do* anything, we hold space in a dynamic way, allowing SelfEmpathy to incubate the healing. We catch our falling wounds by absorbing their momentum and decelerating them. Only then can we hold them in stillness and become whole.

# Forgiveness

You receive forgiveness when you are forgiven and you offer forgiveness when you forgive someone. Forgiving yourself includes both sides because you provide and accept forgiveness. Health and harmony happen when give and take are artfully exchanged, creating the dynamic equilibrium of balanced flow. Like catching yourself, forgiving yourself is an internal interaction where crashed parts of you reconcile and reintegrate into one. Once the wound is caught, it is healed and no longer wounded. It is now healthy. Forgiveness emanates from this place, so you must be whole to genuinely forgive. Your broken parts still in Freeze Flight Fight are unable to Release and make peace. When your TimeLine is healed, you not only let go of your past, you transform the parts of you that suffered.

Empathy converts foe into friend, activating the parasympathetic program of Feed and Breed that nourishes, nurtures, and heals, instructing you to perform helpful and benevolent actions. Instead of "seek and destroy", your parasympathetic side is invested in improving your condition and supporting you in any way possible. Instead of making weapons, you make tools. Aspiring to be helpful comes from a feeling of loving-kindness, a feeling of compassion. This friendly impulse motivates you to do something useful, and forgiveness is profoundly productive. Forgiveness is a deep, parasympathetic instinct that compels you to act with compassion and serve the greater good.

The Trust Fall of Self Healing builds empathy and establishes friendship. Forgiveness redefines foe by absolving everyone unconditionally, which prevents the adrenals from reverting back to stress, discord, and disease. Empathy sets the stage and compassion by converting enemies into allies, merging *other* into *self*. When you successfully catch yourself, your exiled

144

Emothoughts get absorbed. This reboots them and updates the crashed code that created the symptoms in your cells and psyche.

Fallers learn about Release, eventually mastering the 3rd Principle. Experienced catchers Accept and Feel deeply, perfecting the 1st and 2nd Principles. Once you self-heal and become one, you are no longer these two separate characters. The faller gets absorbed into the catcher and this new you is slightly bigger, more skillful, and a bit wiser. This unified you learned lessons and gained invaluable skills when it found the inner strength to befriended its own weakness. Your newly reintegrated self is compassionate: able to forgive and be forgiven. You complete all 3 Principles yourself because the unified you Accepts what happened, Feels it fully, and Releases all of it.

You can't truly forgive if you're still fractured. Your wounded parts in Freeze Flight Fight can't see beyond their reactions. When an angry child is forced to apologize, they avoid direct eye contact and mutter a terse "sorry" that isn't heartfelt. Not ready to Release, they crash and get stuck in false detachment. If you are "trying", you skimmed over the first 2 Principles. When you can't forgive yourself or someone else, repeat the Medical Meditation and absorb that lingering wound. When in doubt, start at the beginning. Catching is Accepting and Feeling, which prepares you for the 3rd and final choice: let go!

The faller has 2 big cathartic moments: stepping off the plank and being safely caught on the other side. These correspond to the 2 phases of the Reboot: unplug and restart. Stepping off the plank unplugs the system from the status quo. When the faller realizes they have been safely caught, they are no longer the old self, the unsafe victim on the plank. The negative experience they had gets neutralized when it gets absorbed into the unified you. It gets redefined because it is no longer helpless and isolated. This is the moment when you actually heal, and the crashed programs regain functional feedback. After your deeply personal trust fall, you restart with an upgrade, gaining skills and wisdom. Pino hopes to go to bed as sticks and strings and awaken as a human child. I don't guarantee that you'll grow an entire nervous system overnight, but you can certainly upgrade your existing infrastructure by Rebooting yourself.

The more you empathize, the more compassion you generate, building your capacity for forgiveness. When you are finally healed and whole, you Release the wounded part of you, surrendering the self that suffered. Because you are at peace, you hold no one to blame for what happened, forgiving everyone involved and moving forward in life.

Becoming a trustworthy catcher awakened your Inner Healer. Now prepare to develop these innate, parasympathetic talents. Your training began with Reboot Camp and culminates with this equally rigorous obstacle course similar to medical school. You will learn advanced skills during these clinical rounds as you are thrust into the fray of alleviating suffering.  You are no longer a *sympathetic soldier* who only attacks or protects; you are now a *parasympathetic peacemaker* tasked with helping those in need. Healers obtain a diagnosis and then provide targeted treatment. In every case, the remedy is the mirror image of the wound, and the Reboot guides you to the core of self-healing: self-reflection.

"To heal thyself, know thyself" implies that self-awareness and accurate introspection activate the Inner Healer. Your built-in tech support comes on-line when you know your networks. When a scientist sets up a clever experiment, they set up a specific environment that reveals how nature operates in that particular circumstance. Illness presents us with a unique challenge and motivates us to pay careful attention to uncover the cure.

# Becoming Medicinal

Forgiveness lets go of your past with grace, elevating empathy into inspired acts of service. Parasympathetic programs are friendly, compassionate, and intrinsically helpful, empowering your cellular physiology, your metabolic Qi machine. Stem cells are master healers because they are programmed to help in any possible way. Stem cells are undifferentiated, which means they have not assumed a specific form. Being amorphous adds the special pixie dust that helps them become the joker, the wild card. Stem cells are flexible enough to become other tissues, making their medicine perfectly suited and tailor-fit to most situations. After your sensory side connects, empathizes, and diagnoses, you deploy your stem cells that become whatever is needed.

## Making New Parts

Our mechanic with a good ear hears how the engine is running and diagnosis the flaw, isolating the faulty part. If they have a replacement part, they can install it and perform the treatment that remedies the problem. If they don't have access to the necessary part, they're out of luck. Unlike a mechanic who fixes cars, a machinist is a specialist that makes parts. Mechanics are like doctors that treat patients in the clinic, doing their best with the tools that they have. A machinist is a researcher that makes parts, building refined tools and crafting better medicines. It takes both sets of skills to heal, just like it takes a village to raise a child.

A common way to make parts is to make a mold and then pour molten steel into it. When the metal cools and hardens, it has the exact shape of the mold. The hot liquid fills the entire space and then solidifies into that specific shape. Dentists make crowns, which are replicas of a tooth, by creating a mold of the original tooth and then pouring in a material that hardens into the replica. A mold is a 3D map of a space, which includes all the contours that define the empty space inside. You attain this accurate map when you connect deeply. When you embody SelfEmpathy, you acquire the blueprints for the mold of the wounded body part. Now that you have the image of the empty mold, your stem cells can fill it and forge themselves into the new part.

Modern machinists also use 3D printers to build specific parts, so rather that pouring liquid into a mold, they program the exact shape and then 3D print the new part. The old-school empty mold that defines the shape gets digitized into the instructions that the 3D printer uses to fabricate the part. Our stem cells are the raw material that gets 3D printed into the healthy version of wounded tissue. This basic idea of a malleable material that can be sculpted into any form is like a sculptor's clay or a wild card that can transform your hand.

The Liquid Trust Fall invokes the property of water enveloping your solid body. My life's work as a manual machinist is focused on transforming my hands into the perfect mold by *feeling into* the tissue. When aqueous hands connect, they wrap around the wound and map it out in 3D. Permission is given and received, trust is established and empathy is attained. This activates the stem cell skills that fill the void the wound created. Sometimes I actually feel the wound sending signals to the brain and then I feel the brain respond by altering the dimmers and reframing how it sees the wound. When the brain befriends the injured tissue, the tissue gets the information it needs to repair itself. This conversation within the self shifts the static, sympathetic compensation to dynamic, parasympathetic collaboration. The adrenal stalemate is broken, and a new path forward presents itself.

Your empathic awareness informs your compassionate stem cell abilities. Your deep insight sparks your ancestral memory, making you nimble enough to become the ideal card. This combined skillset is not just smart, it is wise. Jokers don't just survive tough times, they lighten the mood and offer a helping hand to those who suffer. All wounds need attention, empathy, and care. Once your Inner Healer becomes trustworthy and you befriend your wounds, your parasympathetic programming rebuilds the networks of your mind and body. You update your neural software and upgrade your anatomical hardware.

**Building Pathways**

If you start learning another language, you grow new circuits in your brain to process the new information. The proof is in the pudding, and brain tissue is like custard! The body builds the capacity to handle the load and it grows into its new self. In a similar way, if you hike up hills regularly, you build stronger leg muscles. Like a blacksmith heats metal and pounds it again and again, each hill forges stronger fibers and more resilient fascia. Your lungs will also adjust to the increased demand by capturing more oxygen and injecting it into your blood cells. Bodies also build more arteries and veins in the legs, providing better circulation to fortify the tissue matrix. Your system will do ten thousand things to accomplish the task and meet the challenge. Reboot Camp's Obstacle Course shows us that stress is sometimes necessary to amass strength and advanced skills. Well trained cells gather the tools needed to repair tissues and rebuild neural networks, doing whatever is necessary to meet the demands.

**Forgiveness**

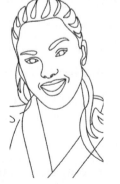

**Liberates You**

In similar fashion, forgiving overcomes the obstacles left from what happened to you. Forgiveness integrates each past impasse into an essential experience. Your traumas and stressors caused you to suffer and forgiveness liberates you from the residue of that suffering. When you see through your reactive, wounded self, and venture beyond your

149

adrenal EmoThinking ego, you become present. You see more of nature. You expand and grow as you extend yourself into this new terrain. As you recognize more of *what is*, you see the bigger picture, and appreciate *all there is*.

Galileo's and Einstein's Thought Experiments led to equations that hold true and reflect natural laws. Accurate awareness augments our abilities to channel natural forces with surgical precision and acquire advanced technologies. When connected and rooted in real-time empathy, your compassionate actions become medicinal. The more you adhere to the 3 Principles, the more potent your medicine becomes. Likewise, when you get ensnared with Freeze Flight Fight, you lose track and dissipate your potential. Forgiveness realigns you with the real events that occurred in your TimeLine so you can live in alignment.

Forgiveness converts would-be traumas into teachable moments you learn from. Forgiving yourself generates internal equilibrium with your past experiences by absolving everyone involved, including you. You don't need to blame others for their transgressions, or punish yourself for your perceived failures and flaws. Forgiveness doesn't make excuses for wrongdoing, condone violence, or ignore the injury that happened. Forgiveness is a willful, conscious choice, and the natural consequence of Accept Feel Release. You take what comes your way, you process it cleanly, and you let go of your experience of that moment. Wounds are especially challenging to process cleanly because our hurt is deeply personal. Once we invest and identify ourself as injured, we latch on to our wound and it defines us. We become the powerless victim on the plank that isn't ready to trust the fall. We take the bait and get ensnared by the simplistic adrenal programming of playing dead, avoiding, or resisting.

Forgive yourself for losing sight of this simple truth when you crash and implode into your adrenal mind, your small self. Others might lose sight of the 3 Principles when they feel threatened, so they'll neglect you or lash out. You'll finally forgive them when you see how their passive-aggressive attacks don't define you or make you a victim. They are just implementing their adrenal programming, so their insults are not personal. Working your way down the adrenal spectrum includes curing chronic EmoThinking. **EmoThoughts don't just turn up dimmers and cause suffering; your EmoThoughts are the parts of you that are actively suffering right now.** Until they are caught and absorbed, they will remain in distress on the plank of their trust fall. As you run stressful scenarios in your mind, you embody these imaginary events and your body physically manifests them. Physical pain is a major factor in people's experience, so EmoThoughts don't create all disease. It's also true that we define most psychological diseases by the EmoThoughts the patient has, like depression, anxiety, panic, paranoia, etc. After decades of treating chronic, intractable pain, I can assert that most pain patients have incessant EmoThoughts *about their pain*. Their condition defines them. In this way, "pain" patients and "psych" patients both define themselves based on how the feel, physically or emotionally. Interestingly, a single neuron can't distinguish physical pain from emotional pain, so a neuron can't really differentiate a broken leg from a broken heart. Neurons just register the hurt; the signal we interpret as pain. Physical pain usually emanates from our anatomy, although not always. While emotional pain also has metabolic roots in chemical imbalance, it's seemingly less physical. Psychological pain seems abstract and *meta*physical, even though it is just as real.

# Water Under The Bridge

Imagine a river out in nature without any signs of people. Settle into a particular part of this river and stay here. Your river can be big or small. It could be a memory of an actual river you visited or an imaginary river.

151

Picture a bridge that crosses the river, and walk halfway across. Look down at the river and watch the water flowing by. Pretend you are holding a rope that has a dozen lumps of cement strung together, so you are standing on the bridge holding this anchor that sinks a bit and gets carried downstream. Get a sense of the river's constant and unrelenting power and feel the resistance of this anchor you are holding. Even if you aren't overpowered by a mighty current, a small river will outlast you. Holding on holds you back, keeping you stuck resisting the flow, testing the river. At some point, whether

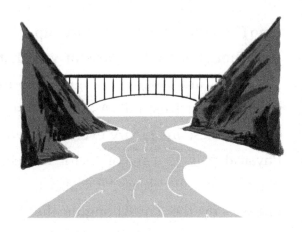

convinced or completely exhausted, you'll let go. Inside each one of these cement lumps is a courtroom scene playing out in your head. There's a prosecutor accusing a defendant of some crime. Depending on your particular EmoThoughts, there are voices blaming someone and another part is being shamed for some flaw. Blame and shame are the name of game, and forgiveness is the only way to win.

The voice that blames and accuses is your Inner Prosecutor. The one being accused is your Inner Defendant. As you might expect, prosecutors embody the Fight response while defendants are in Flight mode. In terms of power, your Inner Defendant is a weak, vulnerable victim and your Inner Prosecutor perpetrates by weaponizing any evidence into accusations. Rather than holding you accountable and helping you atone for your transgressions, this Inner Prosecutor is malicious and seeks punishment.

Listen to your EmoThoughts and distinguish these two characters. What are they saying to each other? Which one of these two characters do you identify with? Which one is YOU? If you blame another person or your circumstances, you are the prosecutor. If you feel bad about yourself, you are the accused. Your Inner Defendant might try to justify itself, providing character witnesses and evidence that they are a good person. Low self-esteem is when your defense council agrees with the accusations, throws in the towel, and concedes that you are a bad seed. Whether you freeze up or fight back, you react to the charges hurled at you. Your Defendant is engaged in the drama and attached to the outcome.

You might feel shame and deep despair. If so, you identify as the defense, and you believe you are that bad person you keep hearing about. Even though you believe you're the Defendant, you are also playing the role of the prosecution. You aren't just the wretched Defendant, you are also the vindictive Prosecutor who is relentlessly making the case against you. To be ashamed, you must be blamed. You might have been mistreated, teased, or bullied in your life, but eventually you internalized that voice and so now it is yours. Perhaps the world gave you the message that you're no good and you believed it. Your EmoThoughts are living out that belief with the endless saga of litigating your worth. It's time to own the fact that you are the one who is accusing you of...whatever accusations you hurl at yourself. That mean voice in your head is also you, even though you might be a nice person who would never hurt someone else. You might love animals and want them to be treated fairly. If you saw someone kick a dog because they were in a bad mood, you would recognize the injustice. Yet many nice folks berate themselves in the privacy of their mind. They might never say mean things to other people but they will dig the knife in when no-one is looking.

**Accountability and Atonement are A-OK**

If your Inner Prosecutor presents evidence of how you behaved poorly, it might be constructive criticism that you can use to improve. In this case, they become your Inner Teacher giving you feedback that helps you. Sincerely own your transgressions and recognize exactly where you crossed the line. Learn from your mistake and accurately confess. Stand accountable with your chin held high. Offer yourself in service and make amends. Humbly ask the court to accept your atonement. You don't want mercy and you are not just apologizing; you want to right the wrong and you are willing to do whatever it takes to help whoever you hurt. Even though this is tough love, it is still love. Your contrition does not emanate from regret, it comes from a proactive impulse to be your best self. You didn't fail, you learned from this teachable moment.

The Intrinsic Breath distinguished assessments from judgments. We welcome any and all assessments, since they provide essential feedback. Judgments, on the other hand, immediately inspire reactions that don't serve the greater good. Judgments are adrenal, short-term reactions and assessments add to our awareness which amplifies our long-term abilities.

Because EmoThoughts are inherently judgmental, they're usually harsh. In these cases your Prosecutor wants vengeance, not accountability. For many people, the jury is like an angry mob with torches and pitchforks ready to punish someone. Listen to your Inner Prosecutor and feel their energy: what is compelling them to bring these charges against you? Are they teaching you or vilifying you? There is only one way to truly know the intentions of this voice: you must step into their shoes and embody the character.

Once you detach from your Inner Defendant enough, you can personify your Inner Prosecutor. Like an actor becoming the character they are playing, study this prosecutor and say their lines with conviction. After all, they fervently believe you should be convicted, and your Inner Defendant is convinced that the charges are real. Good actors embody the energy of their characters, which convinces the audience to suspend disbelief and have a virtual experience through the story. This gives the narrative its power. You might resist playing this role because it can be abusive and mean, but I invite you to really own it. The good news is that once you Accept and Feel, you can Release, detach, and move on, so you are not chained to being this character forever. In fact, if you refuse to Accept and Feel this part of you that blames and accuses, you'll never rid yourself of this critical voice in your head. Your Inner Prosecutor will haunt you and follow you like a shadow until you own the character. We don't transcend our issues, we go through them and transform them. This, in turn, transforms us.

First, you were the beleaguered Defendant and now you're the mean Prosecutor. It's weird but you're playing both sides of the drama. When you EmoThink, figure out which character you identify with and become that character. Then switch and become the other one. Actors train to play different roles, and I'm asking you to be flexible. At any one moment you can feel what the Defendant feels and you can also feel what the Prosecutor feels. When you hold both of these inner characters steady in relative balance, something remarkable occurs.

**This Courtroom Drama Ends Amicably**

Here's the plot twist: you also sit on the bench and wear the judge's robes. You, as the Judge, preside over these proceedings. Your Inner Judge is carefully watching you beat yourself up. It sees that you are the berated, bad one and it also sees the vicious voice who is vengeful and violent. Judges are devoted to justice, and they carry the full authority of the court to uncover the truth. Sit up on the bench, wear the robes, and see through these eyes. From this perspective, your courtroom is a tragic scene, a mockery of the justice system. The evidence is emotional, not factual. The Judge makes the prudent decision to throw out the case and refuses to rule. This wise decision doesn't assign blame or litigate the truth. Dismissing the charges means the Defendant is no longer bound to the accusations. The Defendant is hereby forgiven and free. At this moment, you let go of one of the lumps of cement you were holding against the flow of river.

Forgive yourself. You have the authority. See and feel yourself up on the bench as a wise judge who has presided over many cases and witnessed many scenarios. Hopefully your Inner Defendant feels that it deserves to be forgiven, but even if it doesn't, let it receive forgiveness right now. Like the wounded would-be faller on the plank, this part has felt threatened by harsh accusations. It has been shunned by the community it longs to return to. Fall into forgiveness and Accept the fact that the threat is now cleared. Let this relief wash right through you! When the Judge bangs the gavel and dismisses the case against you, you are no longer the Defendant. Feel the charges fall away. When you are forgiven, you are not right or wrong, so you are not vindicated or castigated. You are free to go on your way without the specter of these accusations following you. These legal charges made you emotionally charged, which disturbed the electrical charges in your brain. Forgiveness is neutrality, so the charges don't stick and they are not attached to you anymore. Forgiveness is an electrical trust fall where you release the electrons that bind you to the negativity of your past.

## Forgiveness Recap

**Step 1:** Notice your EmoThoughts and notice if you are the accuser or the accused. Are you blaming something, or are you being blamed?

**Step 2:** Break out of the character you think you are. You're also the counterpart. Become this other voice and own this other role.

**Step 3:** Hold both parts, recognizing that they're both you. Embody the Inner Prosecutor AND the Inner Defendant.

**Step 4:** Become the Inner Judge: Step onto the bench and wear the robes.

**Step 5:** Dismiss the charges, decline to rule. Forgive your Inner Defendant.

# Forgiveness Debrief

**Forgiveness is releasing an old attachment.** Accepting what happened, regardless of what it was, allows you to Feel and experience what happened, and then Release it. Detachment acknowledges that the past is gone, so the "choice" is to let go. Releasing the past requires processing whatever you are still holding onto, which are the lingering attachments and charges that generate your EmoThoughts. When you actually do the inner work of Accept Feel Release, you unshackle yourself from chronic overthinking. Once liberated, you can now greet your present moment without any reservations or conditions, EmoThought Free!

The word *attachment* has become one of those trendy, new-age words that sounds opaque. What am I really talking about? When 2 things are attached to each other, they are bonded and joined together. You can glue things together or you could sew them together with thread. If you hold on to something, you attach yourself to it as you carry it. Atoms form molecules because opposing charges attract and chemical bonds cement the two atoms into one. The opposite of attachment is detachment, which disconnects the two things that were previously connected. This is why the 3 Principles are arranged in order. When you Accept fully, you open yourself. When you Feel and fully experience the moment you're in, you bond and attach with the experience of that moment. It becomes personal and real for you. Now the trick is to let it go.

Every EmoThought about your past reveals precisely where you are still attached. EmoThoughts might seem like metaphors, but they are literally showing you your issues verbatim. Listen to the words and see the character who is speaking them. When you are tethered to something that already happened, you litigate the past. Judgments remain, and the most important fact is that they are *your* judgments. Other people involved in that past event can be dead and gone, and if you resent what they did or didn't do, you're keeping the event alive, perpetuating it, and dragging it into your HereNow. This keeps you stuck on the bridge holding anchors against the flow of time.

Until you claim these attachments and judgments as your own, you are destined to act out those very same judgments, or their yin/yang opposite, their mirror image. Your behavior will gravitate toward perpetuating that exact crashed loop, or its counterpart. Just like physical symptoms and pain that are telling you something is wrong, your Emothoughts, and the behaviors that they compel you to do, are telling you exactly where they are broken. When they repeat, they are showing you they're crashed. Your BodyMind wants balance, and your EmoThoughts are trying to get your attention. Most people reject their EmoThoughts and wish they would just shut up, but even if they haunt you and drive you nuts, they are your intrinsic self-diagnosis. The Trust Fall of Self Healing introduces you to the prospect that you catch your EmoThinking self to heal your adrenal wounds. Once the wound experiences safety, it has a tangible sense of Friend. Now the voices in your head can tell a new story rather than replay reruns, repeating the same sad saga of samsara and suffering.

## Absolute Value

In math, we have a concept of "absolute value" which we can apply to any number $x$, and by extension, to any experience. We use parallel lines to denote this action of stripping away the plus sign or the minus sign before the number, so all we see is the number itself, the raw value. Plus and minus are conditional, and based on the circumstances the number is in. The absolute value takes the number out of these conditions and just registers the number itself, not the charge that it carries. When your Judge dismisses the charges, forgiveness helps you find the absolute value of each experience. For any number $x$, any experience you have, forgiveness giving you the absolute value. The Forgiveness Function is: $f(x) = |x|$

In physics, charge is an electrical property of particles that we label positive and negative. The reason electrons move through wires is because similar charges repel each other, and opposite charges attract each other. They are compelled to move toward neutral, so they will go toward electrical equilibrium. Electricians call this *ground*, which is the perfect name for it. Raggedy Ann guides us to finding equilibrium in gravity, that we might experience stillness. Forgiveness teaches us to discharge and experience electrical neutrality. Interestingly, the Earth is our source of gravity and it is also the *ground* that absorbs charges.

When lightning strikes, concentrated electrons get projected to the Earth in a giant spark. Why do the electrons leap out of the cloud? They are seeking electrical equilibrium, and the Earth is willing to absorb all those pent-up electrons. It's not because the Earth has a bunch of extra protons that actively pull electrons; it is because there are so, so many atoms that the extra electrons don't really disturb the equilibrium. In the cloud, the electrons are confined next to each other so they are itchy to escape. When the lightning bolt hits the ground, they get integrated and they find a stable home amidst the many, many atoms. Getting grounded is the electrical version of being caught.

Taoism and yin/yang describe equilibrium and recognize that balance is dynamic, not static. A rock on the ground seems still, even though the atoms inside the rock are moving and all of the electrons are zipping around their nuclei at nearly light speed. Electrically, it is not still at all, and each atom's equilibrium is somewhat volatile. The push and pull that repels and attracts charged particles forces them to always move. This perpetual movement sets up changing conditions, so every moment has its own unique equilibrium, depending on where an electron is and where is heading. As particles constantly adapt to changing forces, everything vibrates and oscillates. Flow is the movement of energy that is produced by all of this activity as everything moves toward its equilibrium in its current moment. It sounds poetic to talk about flow, but Taoists have a deep appreciation of this fundamental property of energy exchange. We read the flow patterns and this guides our choices and informs our decisions.

My acupuncture training taught me about The 5 Elements all interact and exchange forces in a dynamic, yet balanced way. Earth represents equilibrium, even though it is revolving around its axis and orbiting the sun. Days are spin cycles and years are circles around the sun. Fire is perpetual action as electrons move, similar to how light vibrates through space. Water is the smooth flow that oscillates back and forth, undulating sine waves. Metal is the atomic structure that holds protons and electrons in close proximity. When atoms stack together and form solids, they can fit together loosely or tightly, and crystals are precisely packed atoms. Wood is life, an organic element. All of this interplay between fire and water, between yin and yang, generates the forces that create the conditions conducive to life. Like fractals and the Fibonacci spiral, there are infinitely many permutations from all of the subatomic variables and quantum fluctuations that are constantly in flux. I'll paraphrase a saying in Taoism that captures this truth: from the yin/yang comes the myriad things, the 10,000 things.

We can also view yin/yang through the lens of attachment and detachment. Anything in your past that repels you (Freeze or Flight) or attracts you (Fight) keeps you tethered to your EmoThoughts that charge you up. Whether you pretend nothing happened, you skip bail, or you zealously re-litigate, these parts of you have *adrenal attachment disorder*. These pent-up charges are static and stuck, like the excess electrons that saturate a cloud and eventually cause stormy weather. Forgiveness harmonizes high voltage electrical pressure, resolving volatility and establishing smooth flow. Now this energy isn't dangerous or caustic, it becomes regulated and useful. Flow makes it friendly, so we can harness it. Luckily, there's an Algorithm of Healthy Flow (the 3 Principles) that you can use to understand and implement this in your life! Attaching is Accepting and Feeling, while detaching is Release. Flow means holding on and letting go fluidly. Flow means catching and falling in a seamless loop, continually exchanging energy and seeking equilibrium. When you get yourself regulated, the 3 Principles repeat by themselves, just like the Earth spins, electrons orbit their nucleus, and clocks tick forward.

The number line in math gives us another way to see how opposites find equilibrium by adding a visual image. Plus and minus represents the duality between a number and its negative counterpart, its mirror image. Each number has an opposing "antinumber" and they always add up to zero. They cancel each other out. The one thing they have in common is their absolute value. I was a math tutor for many years and I translated equations into plain english so math-phobic students could get their bearings and decipher the symbols. The number zero symbolizes neutrality, balance, equilibrium, stillness, peace. The word equivalence has 2 parts, *equi* means equal and *valence* describes electrical charge. Equivalence doesn't just mean equal, it means *electrically* equal. Forgiveness absolves these opposing charges and clarifies your adrenal attachment disorder. To untangle your quantum entanglements, look at your reflection in the quantum mirror.

## Here's a Question: Authority?

Authority is a position of power. Your orders are obeyed. If you have authority, you claim the mantle of being an author and dictating what happens. You pick up a pen to write narratives and the characters in the stories have no choice but to say their lines and act out the script they are given, implementing the writer's decree. You are the author of your own story, and you define the rules of the road for yourself. Pino wants to be in charge of his bones, so his trust fall invited you to reclaim your dimmers. Your catcher takes charge and guarantees the safety of the faller, which awakens your Inner Healer. Your Inner Judge is charged with the authority to preside over the proceedings and cleanly process past events. Are you ready to claim your power, clean up your mental courtroom, and discharge your EmoThoughts?

You need to see both sides of the warring factions within yourself to claim authority and become the Inner Judge. Become an independent witness as the two sides hash out their conflicting perspectives about the truth. To become trustworthy, don't play favorites. The innocent Defendant must stand firm and a guilty Defendant must atone. The Prosecution has the right to accuse, but they are officers of court and must abide by the rules, or else they lose their privileges to stand before the judge. They can hold a guilty person accountable, but they must be dispassionate as they provide this essential feedback. If the same EmoThoughts persist after you forgive yourself, you'll need to go back and do it again. Only this time, be more specific and more convincing. If you identify as a victim, being the Defendant is easy, since you've had tons of practice. Step into the Prosecutor's role and say those lines with all of your energy. Give your best performance, the version the director puts in the movie. Your Reboot Drill Sergeant is now your acting coach, preparing you to convince the most skeptical audience: you!

You might bounce around between accuser and accused for a while before you dare step up on the bench and be the Judge. You don't have as many lines as the other two characters, but everything you say is grounded with conviction. You hold the authority because you represent the pursuit of truth and jurisprudence. To really embody the Judge, conjure the feeling of empowered command that is earned through deep knowing. From this position of power, the Judge is tasked with being impartial, and truly open. Authority comes from the commitment to being humble, selfless, and nonjudgmental. It's ironic! Blamers and shamers are tangled up in a spiral of suffering and the Judge is there to sort it all out with clarity.

Part of the prosecutors power comes from an all-out assault, attacking and accusing in a blitzkrieg of charges. Your Judge's power is different. The source isn't fervor or emotion, it's temperance. The Judge has vision: the ability to see all sides of an issue and arrive at justice. It is your sovereign right to claim the authority to preside over your EmoThinking mind and restore order into your mental courtroom.

Once you establish this authority, you are in charge of your mind. If any voices challenge the Inner Judge's dominion over the courtroom, look them in the eye and exert soft power. Rather than yell or ask the bailiff to remove them, win an Oscar by speaking directly to the Inner Prosecutor who is out of line. Be professional and embody the authority of the bench upon which you sit. Connect on a human level and show them that you acknowledge their argument and that you value their version of the truth, even though you are overruling them.

# Here Comes

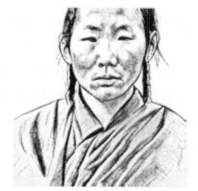

# The Judge

When the catcher sees the faller with empathic eyes, the faller feels trust and gains permission to let go. The judge also connects, but rather than projecting trustworthiness, they exude authority. Like parenting a child who is throwing a tantrum, we need to keep our cool, listen respectfully and let them vent while holding the boundary firm. We don't accept their abusive outbursts while simultaneously recognizing their imbalance and feeling compassion for their suffering. Once they feel seen and heard (and their blood sugar regulates), they stop acting out. Holding this supple yet firm boundary provides the space for them to work out their internal angst and find calm. When you preside over your mind in this way, you create a platform that allows your EmoThoughts to self-regulate and find their resolution, their personal equilibrium. They are just reacting to their circumstances, and you can help them arrive at the permission they need to stop accusing, defending, litigating, resisting, and fighting. Like your Inner Healer that catches, the Judge is safe and secure. They aren't in Freeze Flight Fight, which means they aren't traumatized, defensive, or aggressive. They are balanced and poised, proficient and powerful. Put on your judicial robes and emerge from your chambers to preside over your courtroom: "All rise, order in the court."

## Converting Vicious Cycles into Compassion Cycles

When a vicious cycle spins in the other direction it becomes a compassion cycle. Instead of circling the drain and getting sucked down the vortex into the abyss, when you spin in the other direction you come up the cone, expanding into a bigger space. Instead of paying interest that gets compounded into your debt, your dividends get reinvested and profits multiply exponentially. All of the negative energy that weighed you down becomes empowering and elevates you. Healing converts wounds into lessons, transforming liabilities into capabilities. Ask any drug counsellor who was an addict and you'll hear their story about how their wound became their medicine. They did the inner work that converted their weakness into their strength, and in the process they gained insights as they learned tough life lessons.

Compassion isn't just flowery talk about flow. Forgiveness understands suffering intimately because you must Accept and Feel before you Release. We don't transcend, we go through. You faced an obstacle and you met the challenge without a guarantee that it will be all roses forever and ever. The peace was earned and it isn't permanent because as conditions change, our equilibrium needs to be adjusted. Clearing the static charges from all of the repetitive EmoThoughts breaks up the storm clouds so the sun can shine through. When you reconcile all of the voices, they quiet down and you experience a state of deep peace. Settling into this feeling helps you realize you don't need to think all the time and you don't need to crank up your dimmers. You are just fine without chaos. Not only are you ok, you can channel your energy toward your health, or you can help others.

**Receive Forgiveness: Bask in the Light**

Let your Inner Defendant stand before the Judge and be absolved of all charges! Give all of these negative charges to the Earth, which can absorb them all. Let your Defendant feel the exaltation of being cleansed from the doubts that cloaked their absolute value. As the charges fall off, your suffering and your shame also wash away. Kneel or lie down and allow your Inner Defendant to receive this gift. Weep in gratitude as this loving energy blasts through you like x-rays, melting the sticky, tar-like residue of your somatized attachments. Any dark, shadowy places get illuminated and your Inner Defendant is no longer a powerless victim who is flawed or bad. The Reboot challenges you to relax all the way and Forgiveness challenges you to fully experience the bliss of being truly free.

Try this Thoughtless Experiment: Put the book down, lay your body down on the ground, and discharge all of the pent-up negative charges you have been carrying and attached to. Give them to the Earth and get grounded. After you discharge, you'll get recharged…

## Relative and Absolute

Your personal experience is relative to your conditions. Forgiveness is unconditional, which means forgiveness is absolute. It doesn't depend on what happened, who did what, who got hurt, or how they got hurt. We Accept that it happened, we Feel and connect to the experience of what happened, as horrible as it may be. We don't just feel our own pain, we also empathize with everyone's personal experience. Then, we Release all of the attachments we have. This liberates us from what occurred, and it also gives others an offramp to discharge their attraction or repulsion that binds them to the past.

Our experiences don't define us. It's true that profound experiences alter us, but we don't have to carry them with us. Moments pass *through* us, but they are not who and what we are. We are the processor of moments, so we are not the moments that we process. Book 2 describes presence as a camera that registers what occurs. If you are the camera, you are not the pictures you take. You are vessel that processes each photograph, recording each moment in time. Your memories aren't just visual images; your body is a somatic camera that biochemically stamps experiences into your tissues.

It's tricky to ascertain the intrinsic truth. It's hard enough to let go of yourself enough, so you can experience your Intrinsic Breath. The next 60 pages help you unpack the subtle layers of your adrenal mind that ignores what is, avoids what is, or resists what is. In keeping with the 3 Principles motif, you're invited to actively Accept, proactively Feel, and deliberately Release any narrative about what happened.

# Forgiveness 2.0

## Intro to the Outro

These 3 subchapters reapply the 3 Principles so you can fully forgive yourself, forgive others, and be forgiven. We unfreeze by waking up to the subliminal, we bravely experience all of the parts of ourself, and then we let go of our story.

1) Accept - Stenographer records self talk —> Script and characters.
2) Feel - Act out EmoThoughts —> Embody each character. Somatics.
3) Release - Write a new story —> Create new narrative, new characters.

Step 1 is to Accept your subliminal script: journal and write down EmoThoughts. A stenographer records what was said and identifies who said it, which defines the characters. They don't interpret the script; they just listen and accurately record everything.

Step 2 is to Feel and act out each character that is EmoThinking. Empathize. Believe you are them, assume their identity, and embody their energy. Feeling is somatic. *Embody their understanding.* Internalize the experience and live out the moment.

Step 3 is to Release and rewrite. You already lived that old story and there is nothing left for you to learn from it. Write a new narrative, invent new characters, and create your new future. Dare to live an unscripted improv!

# ACCEPT: THE STENOGRAPHER

## Accepting What Is

become aware of everything you buried
behind walls you built in your mind
protecting and insulating you
from harsh weather

beyond forgiveness lies a conscious witness
an ear that clearly hears
the self-talk rattling around in your brain
recording your subliminal script

write it down, make it known
bring the unconscious into conscious awareness
the stenographer has no skin in the game
of litigating truth

-Poet Zero

If you truly want to dismantle stress and heal deeply, you will need to examine all the EmoThoughts that inflame your cells and compel you to turn up your dimmers. A thorough dissection of your EmoThoughts yields a detailed diagnosis of crashed loops in your neural software.

Question:    How do we arrive at this deeper self-awareness?
Answer:    Write down all of your EmoThoughts.

Record the voices echoing through your head by writing down the words you hear in your brain. Journaling is the lab report of your mind. An MRI image shows where your tissues are compromised and bloodwork reveals physiological imbalance. Like physical pain, your EmoThoughts are symptoms, expressions of imbalance that are attempting to alert you that something is amiss. When you think the same thoughts over and over, you are in a crashed loop of chronic emotions and tangled mental energy.

A stenographer in a courtroom records everything people say, so every word that is spoken gets written down. Get a pen and paper and become the stenographer that records your EmoThoughts, or speak them into a recorder if you prefer. Don't edit or judge what you hear, just write it all down or say it out loud. Don't short-change yourself by filtering and avoiding your harshest EmoThoughts. Write them all down, even if you would rather skip the nasty rhetoric you might hear when it is quiet and you are all alone.

You don't need to share your secrets with anyone. I only ask that you confess to yourself. Acceptance involves becoming aware, which is deeply personal. Noone else needs to know your inner truth, but my clinical experience clearly shows that you must be connected to yourself to be healthy and powerful. If you dare to become aware of the subliminal script in your mind, you might be tempted to gloss over certain EmoThoughts and shield yourself. Flight avoids Feeling and keeps you stuck at the 2nd Principle. If you're ashamed for having nasty EmoThoughts, your Inner Prosecutor is accusing you. The only way out of this crashed quagmire is to forgive yourself for having harsh EmoThoughts. How can judging yourself harshly for being harsh make you less harsh? Converting judgments into assessments opens you to Accepting your internal discord, so you finally see it for what it is. Without the overlay of good or bad, you have a chance to clarify your wounded, adrenal characters that are vying for a safe place in your mind and body.

## Discovering Your Inner Stenographer
## An 8 Minute EmoThought Experiment

1) Set a timer for 2 minutes.
2) Write down every word you hear in your brain.
3) When the timer rings, set another 2 minute timer.
4) Read the words you wrote down in the first 2 minutes.
5) Your journal is a script: Identify the characters and name the voices.
6) When the timer rings, set another 2 minute timer.
7) Say each character's lines out loud, like an actor playing that role.
8) When the timer rings, set another 2 minute timer.
9) Sit quietly and contemplate. Who are the various characters that are EmoThinking in your mind? Who is the stenographer that wrote their words down? Who read those words aloud? Who is now contemplating the script of your self-talk?

When the final timer rings, you can store this journal entry for reference or shred it. You can also safely burn it and bury the ashes in the dirt, using the fire to convert the words on the paper to ash and then putting them in the ground. The Earth can absorb all of your secrets, your subliminal fear, your rancor, your entire shadow side. Notice your breath. Watch the balloon fill with air and use your exhale to let go any emotions or attachments.

Did you discover any new characters lurking around in your subconscious? Did you learn more details about familiar characters like your Inner Defendant or your Inner Prosecutor? You might have heard about the Inner Child, the part of you that is innocent and open to the world. This part isn't ashamed or bored, but rather in a state of wonder about the mysterious world. My personal internal research also revealed an oppositional voice that reflexively resists and rebels, whom I call my Inner Teenager. There are also the traumatized parts that are frozen. One patient described "the girl in the doorway" as a terrified child who stands frozen while her parents fight. She doesn't speak, so she might be hard to recognize, yet her persona represents a juvenile part of you that is overwhelmed. Another important persona is the Inner Protector, something or someone that protects the Inner Child. It could be a wolf, a warrior, a dragon, or a kindergarten teacher. This persona will never harm the Inner Child and they will do anything to keep the child safe. Unlike the adrenals that often stifle us in the name of safety, the Inner Protector isn't overbearing, so the child remains free to play and daydream. However, if anyone encroaches and threatens this innocent child, the Protector will pounce and repel the attack.

As a medical practitioner, I don't need to know everything about my patients, I only need to recognize their crashed loops and their strengths. I ask a lot from myself because I aspire to see them as they are and to accurately reflect their energy back to them, so they can reconcile their turbulence and reestablish flow. Patients, and you the reader, are also given a big task: go inwardly and Accept everything you encounter. Later, when you Feel it all and Release it, you Reboot and restore function to your metabolic Qi Machine. Before we get into the trenches and do the nitty gritty work of self-healing, we must get our bearings and get centered in reality. Acceptance comes first. You will process the material that you are unearthing in due time. Your stenographer is the part of you that Accepts, full stop. There's no Feeling or Releasing involved. Stenographers don't have time to process the script; their mission is to keep listening to the dialogue so they don't miss anything.

Reboot Camp trains you to unplug your reactive motor side and become a sensory soldier, a sentient sentinel who is on the front line of what's actually happening, aka *what is*. The first skill is to separate sensory from motor, distinguishing perceiving from doing. If you decline doing and you dive into your sensory side, you Accept the data coming toward your brain. Opening the sensory side is Accepting reality by letting $x$ be $x$, regardless of what $x$ is. Like a hidden video camera, your stenographer takes it all in. In the same way the Intrinsic Breath invites you to get out of the way and witness your body breathe all by itself, your stenographer watches your mind as it EmoThinks. All of the dialogue your stenographer records is objective, unvarnished, and accurate. To access this highly refined state, you must fully commit to the sensory side and become the passive witness.

Water Under The Bridge asked you to be the Defendant and the Prosecutor in equal measure, so that you can embody a new and powerful character: the Judge. While the Judge has the authority to rule, the Stenographer has a unique perspective which gives them special powers. Because they don't have skin in the game, they never speak and they don't play a role in what occurs. They are a silent witness who only listens. They hear everything and record it. They don't process or interpret anything that is said, so they have no opinions, judgments, or assessments about the case. They are not threatened by anything, so they have no adrenal reaction. Because they are detached, they have no need to Feel, which empowers them to simply Accept. If they were to digest what happens, they would get distracted by their internal process and they would miss something. Their script would have gaps, like blind spots. They have a simple yet solemn role: document the events that are transpiring.

Stenographers take their job seriously, and their diligence offers many gifts. Their vital service produces the official record, an accurate transcript. Unlike a microphone that just registers the words that are spoken, the stenographer's record also includes the names of the various people that are speaking. This provides a framework that helps us understand the dialogue and envision the scene. The official record looks exactly like a movie script, which is the template actors use to say their lines and act out their part. Labelling the voices **defines the characters** and transforms a raw transcript into a tangible script that tells an important story. Naming the characters is a huge asset because it helps us relate to what our characters have gone through and how they feel, deep down inside. Listening to self-talk without distinguishing who is saying each line keeps the EmoThoughts jumbled and unintelligible, so you can't gain a foothold or traction to unpack the issues.

Our EmoThinking characters fall into 3 familiar categories: traumatized personas in the freezer, defensive voices deflecting accusations, and fighters that blame someone. Anytime you become aware of an adrenal EmoThought, ask yourself if it's frozen, flighty, or aggressive. Your stenographer training involves clearly identifying each character, but before you try naming them, find out which phase of the 3Fs they are in. The Reboot Camp Obstacle Course teaches you to get a grip and a foothold, so you can climb the slippery wall. Get a gist of who this character is by sensing how they Feel. As the stenographer, you don't empathize, you simply register how they Feel. Clearly naming the voices helps you understand their survival concerns and core motivation. This enables you to scale the wall that separates the wounded parts of you from your heart.

The Stenographer's service is to Accept every voice in your mind and identify who they are. Acceptance requires a singular mindset and a high degree of discipline: remain laser focused on the *ear that hears*. No distractions! Any temptation to Feel what the speaker is projecting pulls the ear away from the next words. It's hard to stay this focused and resist being drawn into the drama, but this is required if you want to unearth everything that has been buried. Physical pain presents us with a similar challenge that tests our discipline. When a sensory signal hits the brain and gets decoded as pain, it is very tempting to react by blocking it. At that moment, we stop listening and we insulate ourselves, or we fight it by wanting to change it and remove it. When the next pain signal arrives at the brain a second later, we are less able to work with it because we are ignoring it, minimizing it, or resisting what is.

In the Trust Fall of Self Healing I said catching includes Accepting and Feeling. Accepting recognizes the faller and Feeling absorbs the momentum of the falling body. I said Accepting is unconditional and somewhat impersonal, saying that the Earth will always Accept you when you fall, but rocks don't cushion your landing. For now, stay detached and don't Feel. Don't fall for Feeling and get enmeshed with wounded fallers. Instead, focus on recognizing that there is an EmoThought on the plank and name the persona inside the bubble. Another part of you will Feel and absorb that faller when they are ready to jump. Before the Inner Healer can empathize and catch a faller, they have to clearly recognize them up on the plank. The Stenographer registers the EmoThinking voice and names it. In fact, a good stenographer defines every character by training themselves to reject all filters and bias, so they can Accept everyone unconditionally.

The Medical Meditation emphasizes Feeling as the part of your Inner Healer that befriends the EmoThought in the bubble and brings them back into your heart. I described a fiber optic cable that connects your wound to your heart center. I asked you to hold your empathic attention steady to build the bandwidth of this 2-way cable that enables a dialogue between you and the wound. Acceptance is the first thread that links your parasympathetic skills with your sympathetic, adrenal wounds. Without Acceptance, the empathic part of you would remain blind and oblivious to the wounded EmoThoughts trapped inside the bubble. Your empathic skills are useless if you don't have a character to relate to. How can you walk in someone else's shoes if you don't even see them, recognize who they are, and truly know that person? Empathy doesn't just happen; before you Feel, you must Accept.

Accepting again and again adds more filaments to your cable, strengthening the bond between the faller and the catcher. This thicker cable not only allows the catcher to see who is trapped inside the bubble, it also allows the faller to register your kind-hearted attention. Realizing they have been seen and recognized alters the suspicious faller, which makes them feel safer. When the catcher sees the faller soften a tiny bit, they recognize that fact and Accept them as they are now. When the catcher Accepts continuously, they bond with the faller in real time, which is when Feeling begins.

To understand how Acceptance becomes Feeling, imagine how individual pixels get compiled into a composite image that has more meaning than any one dot. One drop of ink doesn't paint a clear picture, and it takes many pixels to create a photograph. When you keep Accepting each moment, each individual data point gets plotted on a graph and a novel shape emerges. Arranging all of the factoids reveals a pattern, which is why the whole is greater than the sum of the parts. Acceptance amasses accurate data, while Feeling graphs the pixelated personality traits and creates a multifaceted character with a story to tell. Our hero/heroine has been through the school of hard knocks and is wounded by the world. How does their story end? Are they redeemed? Do they reconcile their wounds and teach us how to navigate our own life?

My definition of cognition is to become aware, which boils down to processing a sensory signal. If a sensor gets triggered, it sends a signal to your brain. When your brain decodes it, in whatever way it can, you become cognizant of the sensation. You see light, smell garbage, hear a bell ring, taste food, or somatically Feel pleasure or pain. If you reapply your attention to the current signals

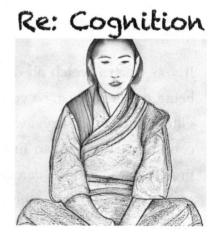

**Re: Cognition**

coming from your sensors, and you process them without bias or judgment, you get meta-data. Cognition is being aware of a single sensory signal, whereas recognition is being aware of a multitude of signals that keep coming in every millisecond. As you collate and assemble the flood of data from your body, moment by moment, you don't just become more aware, you build nuanced self-awareness. Acceptance becomes Feeling when impersonal data becomes your very personal experience, and gets encoded as a frame in your filmstrip, your TimeLine.

## Breaking the Ice

Your Stenographer thaws out your frozen, traumatized parts. They are willing to Accept the fact that you buried intense experiences because you were overwhelmed. Your system couldn't take it in so you did what you needed to do to survive that moment, which means building a wall to keep that experience at bay. Your stenographer is antifreeze, and they don't judge you for shutting down. Since Freeze is a dissociative state of being disconnected, breaking the ice accurately describes cutting through the frozen crust to establish contact. In social situations we also *break the ice* by saying hello, offering a handshake, or bowing to acknowledge the other person. This Accepts and recognizes the other's presence, which opens the door to connecting and conversing. Namaste!

### Is Ignorance Willful?

If you wear a watch all day, you acclimate and ignore the sensation of it being on your wrist, so you can focus on more important, realtime events. Filtering our sensory awareness helps us prioritize where we put our conscious attention, so that we can engage in the right way at the right time. Overdeveloped *adrenal awareness filters* block important information and insulate us from the real world too much, locking us in our own bubble.

Confirmation bias is a term that describes how we selectively ignore anything that might contradict our perspective. We also seek information that reinforces our beliefs. Following the Friend or Foe playbook of adrenal survival, our bubble is calibrated to block threats and to Accept reinforcement. EmoThoughts feed the Foe mentality and play a major role in determining what gets through and what remains ignored. Repetitive and crashed EmoThought loops harden the filter and double down on blocking anything deemed as *other*. We get rigid as we habituate over time. Our mental inertia makes our bubble thick with the haze of neural static and we lithify into our own prejudice.

It's tricky to find the balance between being hyperaware of every little thing and living in a bubble. We can find insight in the unlikely example of modern garage floodlights that have a motion sensor. Adding the motion sensor makes the light more efficient and saves power because it activates only when there is a need. Rather than leaving the light on all night and wasting energy for no reason, the motion sensor perceives movement, which then sends current to the bulb to turn it on. Like our nervous system, the sensor is connected to a switch, so when the adrenals are triggered, there's an automated response that sends current to muscles and the EmoThinking mind. This raises an important question: "how do you calibrate your sensors that recognize things?" When a garage light is too sensitive, it is too easily triggered. When the sensor gets numb and can't register a person walking by, it also needs to be updated and recalibrated.

The Reboot not only shuts off the motor system for a time, Rebooting also recalibrates your sensory system so that you can detect pertinent information. Your Stenographer has a sophisticated *EmoThought detector* that hears the subliminal script in your head. If your EmoThoughts are beneath your conscious awareness, you become like a floodlight with a broken sensor that never registers movement, and remains in darkness. If you filter and block your harsh thoughts and emotions, you are keeping yourself in Freeze Mode. Those emotions are still buried behind walls in your mind that keep them hidden and out of sight. The partition in your mental hard drive blocks your conscious awareness, so you are not just helpless, you become hapless. Before you break through these walls you made to insulate yourself, you must simply recognize them and Accept the fact that the walls are there. Checking your bias calibrates your sensory side so you recognize what you might have previously ignored.

## Beyond Bias: Expanding Your Range

Look in the mirror. What do you see? Ask yourself if you are willing to remove your blinders. It's ok if you are unwilling. Just admit it and forgive yourself for now. You kinda know you are biased, but you acclimated to your new normal that chooses to not see it. You didn't really investigate or look into it. You have the excuse that you were unaware, that it was out of your purview, and that you were not obliged to dig deeper and find out what might be hidden behind door number 3. After all, some things are out of our grasp. My eyes don't detect infrared light, so I have no physical way of knowing that this light is all around me. I know it is there from an academic perspective, but I don't have the sensory capacity to see it with my own eyes. If you are in a dysfunctional relationship, it might seem easier to ignore the problems because it feels overwhelming to face the facts and act accordingly. As Cat Stevens said, "it's hard, but it's harder to ignore it." The strategy of Freeze keeps it buried, but eventually reality wins because $x=x$, whether you Accept the truth or not.

Here's a silly anecdote to illustrate how we selectively ignore things we don't want to see. When my daughter was young, she sometimes had a messy room with clothes scattered on the floor. One day she tossed a T-shirt on the kitchen floor and left it there. Instead of picking it up, I left it there. A while later, when she walked through the kitchen, I asked her to pick it up and deal with it. She immediately and emphatically said that she didn't see it. She was genuine and sincere, even though our kitchen isn't that big and the shirt was in the way, so she had to step over it. I was tempted to confront her with the fact that the shirt was an obstacle, which includes a litany about what she "should" do, etc. Instead I asked: "if that shirt was a one hundred dollar bill on the floor, do you think you would have noticed it?" She stopped in her tracks and realized that she would have noticed a shiny object. Her facial expression and body language revealed that she was busted, bless her heart! At that moment she grappled with her choice to ignore the shirt because it didn't have value, and that she would have bothered to see money on the kitchen floor.

After a few moments, my next comment was, "you probably would have bent down to pick it up." In the same way a motion sensor turns on the light, seeing money on the floor turns on the motor side to pick it up. Because putting a shirt in the hamper is boring, the easiest way to avoid the chore is to subconsciously ignore that it exists. I had my own epiphany about the profound gravity of unconscious bias as a 10-year old, the first time I truly heard this Paul Simon lyric: "Still a man hears what he wants to hear and disregards the rest." I knew in my bones that I was also susceptible to this flaw, and these words whisper in my ear from time to time. The Freeze defense pretends the Emperor has no clothes, which begs the question: "what are you willing to see?"

Another way to ask this question is, "what are willing to ignore, and sweep under the rug?" Your Stenographer Accepts unconditionally and looks under the rug. The Stenographer hears the voices buried in the basement, behind the walls you built to protect yourself from harm or taking responsibility. Your Stenographer is tasked with bringing all of the skeletons out of your closet and writing out their stories. Odds are, there's a pile of dirty laundry in your BodyMind, and you might be tiptoeing around it and pretending it's not there. Because unprocessed content gets stored and buried in your organs and tissues, your Stenographer is also an archeologist. When I palpate a patient's body, I feel some of the material that is stored in the tissue, and this catalyzes their Trust Fall of Self Healing.

Even though your impersonal and impartial Stenographer only listens, they speak for your most beleaguered and traumatized personas. They don't promise to Feel or empathize, they just recognize them and make their voices heard by recording them, so you can't pretend they don't exist. Acknowledgement is the first step toward trust, and Acceptance is the first hurdle on the road to becoming trustworthy. Your Inner Healer catches fallers with both devotion and skill. Acceptance is devotion and Feeling is skill. Put your skills on the shelf for now and ask your heart to perceive something that's right under your nose.

In a fundamental way, the question of *willingness* can be restated as: how much healing do you really want? How much truth can you handle? How much of yourself are you willing to catch? Are you ready to own it and walk your talk, or are you going to play lip service to your deepest truth? We all make own own choices, and we live and die by the consequences. When a patient lays down on my treatment table, I reflect their wounded energy back to them, so they can process it and *make sense* of it. In my role as a healer, I'm just a mirror. Like the Hubble telescope, my job is to polish my mirror so I can reflect a clear image and give my patient's body and mind the information it needs to see itself in its totality. This clear diagnosis Reboots crashed loops and restores feedback to the neural software. The updated parasympathetic system upgrades the anatomical hardware, recasting new parts and weaving new tissue to optimize your biochemical and mechanical human Qi Machine.

## Who's Who

Of all the characters in this courtroom, who is the most important? You might identify as the Defendant which makes this character real for you.

You might choose the Judge, since they have authority to rule. Sometimes defense attorneys use affirmations and compelling character references to affirm a positive self-image that rebukes the accusations, so you might nominate them as the most important person. The Prosecutor plays a prominent role, since they create the drama by accusing the accused. I believe the most important character is the Stenographer. Why? They are fully aware of everything, with their sensory side open, yet they are not one of the actors. If you're busy pleading for mercy or wanting to punish, you're still *in* the drama. Even forgiving yourself is dramatic. When you step away from the motley crew of characters and their personal experiences, you can see the whole scene unfold.

The Stenographer personifies Acceptance because they agree to not get distracted by processing the dialogue they hear. They have no skin in the game, so they steadfastly Accept whatever happens. If your skin has scars, your adrenal mind will jump in and protect you by selectively ignoring anything that caused you to suffer. Stenographers aren't just born with this acute awareness; they acquire this ability by strictly adhering to the 3rd Principle of Release. Acceptance doesn't just happen; it is the product of Releasing everything else that came before, so the Zen Beginner's Mind can perceive what is. The 3 Principles are circular, so the more you let go, the more you Accept, and your Stenographer accrues more awareness.

When you see that you aren't any one of these characters, you realize how you're really all of the characters. Stenographers don't have the luxury to litigate these characters because they are deeply devoted to seeing them interact and witnessing what is. Forgiveness diffuses the emotional fuse that drives each persona, allowing you to detach form all of them. Rather than bouncing around from one character to the next, when you no longer identify as the actors, you can follow the storyline as the courtroom drama plays out. Because you are simultaneously all of the characters and none of them, you are something else entirely.…

# FEEL: Actors Embody Emotion

## Somatic Stories

Stories suspend disbelief
audiences dare to believe
dare to feel the experiences
the actors embody

empathize with your emothoughts
enact their stories
own your somatic script
to create a new narrative

beliefs drive emothoughts
emothoughts drive behavior
believe it or not
believemothoughts are what you manifest

-poet zero

Stop reacting and act. Actors generate actions. Their energy activates empathy and induces experiences in the audience, inspiring internal events in their biochemistry. Fictional stories and playing make-believe become real when the audience Feels. Touched by the events they vicariously lived through, they do things and exert forces in the real world.

**-Bea Eniwun**, Reboot Acting Coach

Earlier today while treating a patient, I felt a blockage in the base of her skull and upper neck. I used my hands to feel into the tissue which attracts me toward the tension. Once I find the glitch, I wrap my hands around it and hold it. Soon enough, the brain realizes I'm there and it responds to my precise touch. This patient realized that she was unable to let go, and she tried to relax as I focussed on the stubborn issue. Within moments she remarked that she was remembering an event from years ago that she hadn't thought of recently. She thought she had resolved that issue but she was reminded that her body still held some residue.

She asked me if I was reading her mind and I replied that I was reading her body. While it is true that I had images about what happened, it is not my business to get involved with the details of the event she was remembering. My sole purpose for tapping into this place is to show her the unresolved content so that *she* can process it. My hands are like a stenographer that hears the rumblings within the tissues and when I *listen into* the system, I unEarth lingering aspects of whatever was stored in the body. The brain is then presented with this unresolved stuff, and memories often pop into their awareness. When I feel the brain connect to the somatic content, I maintain my neutral presence so that the mind can receive the memories that were stored in the body. This gives both the mind and the body the space to Accept Feel Release whatever needs to get ingested, digested, and excreted.

This chapter delves into the physical body which has its own language, and words are not part of this somatic syntax. When unprocessed experiences get stored in the tissues, they get translated into this anatomical dialect which is not tangible to the brain. By the same token, when these stored moments in the body's basement are recognized by the brain, they get converted into something tangible, like sensations, thoughts, emotions, and dream-like images. They come back into the purview of the 5 senses, so they can finally get processed cognitively. This fascinating interplay between the body's somatic perspective and mind's psychological linguistics is explored in granular detail in the Book 2 of The Quantum Needle Trilogy. We can simplify for now and say: the mind expresses itself through EmoThoughts and behavior, while the body communicates with pain, inflammation, tissue restriction, and organ dysfunction.

Now it's your turn to step up by healing yourself. Hippocrates is famous for saying: "Physician, heal thyself." Your first and most important patient is you. Your EmoThoughts are in need, and they're telling you exactly where they are stuck. Your physical body is also telling you it is faltering when it hurts, gets stiff, fatigued, or weak. Accepting makes you aware, and Feeling translates these signals into actionable intelligence.

## The Body Is A Battery

Batteries store energy. A typical battery holds lots of electrons which can be used to power a phone or an electric car. A mousetrap is a non-electrical battery that stores mechanical energy in the coiled spring. Your body is a complex battery that stores moments that overwhelmed you because **unprocessed experiences get stored in the tissues**. After a fall, your fascia holds the mechanical energy from the impact. Your fascia also holds emotional energy from impactful experiences. Terms like *muscle memory* are useful, but the bulk of the memory is stored in the nervous system, not in the muscle tissue. The nervous system sends the current that tells muscles what to do, so muscles are less conscious than the nerves that control them. Muscles follow the commands of the dimmers, like Pinocchio's strings that are pulled by the puppeteer's hand. Organs like the liver, kidneys, and pancreas experience emotion much more than muscles do. We associate love with the heart, which is not a mistake, because the vital organs Feel everything keenly. In this context, organs and the neural system store more emotional energy than muscles, so they are better batteries.

Both acupuncture and Visceral Manipulation help the body redistribute pent-up energy, whether from mechanical or emotional trauma. We use the term *compensation* to describe how we adapt to an injury, like limping after hurting your ankle. Putting more weight on your good leg sets up a pattern of muscular imbalance. Even after your injured ankle heals, the muscles often continue to fire asymmetrically. Interestingly, the body has the same muscles on the right and left side, so you have a right tricep and a left tricep. Sometimes, I picture the dimmer console in the brain arranged with these right-left pairs. If one dimmer switch is higher than its counterpart, the muscle on that side will be shorter, and your skeleton will be pulled out of whack. Every patient has some degree of compensation in their body, whether from injuries, overuse, or sitting too much. I also see similar physical effects from emotional compensation too. Childhood trauma can leave a deep imprint in the nervous system which makes it very hard for people to trust they are safe. Even when people are alone and safe in their own bed, they often feel anxious and turn up their dimmers. When you EmoThink, your neural software is limping and struggling to get by. The meditations in this book are specific treatments that de-compensate you, releasing the old patterns that helped you survive in the short-term, but hamper you in the long run. Forgiveness discharges the charges and the stagnant Qi, so your system runs smooth with less inflammation.

Your Stenographer serves as a catalyst by recognizing unresolved content. Listen to it and *Feel into it,* so the brain can Accept Feel Release. This sets up a dialogue within the self where the wound can be seen, then caught and absorbed. Every day in my clinic I preside over this process and facilitate the 3 Principles: I Accept and unearth the stored charges, I coach the system to Feel into itself and process those charges. When the system catches itself and integrates the disconnected wounds, I invite the system to Release all of it. This cleanses and reorganizes the body and the mind, harmonizing the mental software with the somatic hardware. Jean Pierre Barral taught me and countless others to manually listen to the body with precision and acuity. I also teach therapists how to manually listen to organs, nerves, and fascia. This book teaches you how to listen to yourself.

To study human nature, take a look at how babies process the world. Do you remember the Reboot Rock-a-Bye? How do we communicate to a baby that it is ok for them to surrender into sleep? We cradle them, we rhythmically rock them, and we might hum a lullaby. In a similar way, the back of your breathing balloon rhythmically massages your adrenals and comforts the part of you in Freeze Fight Fight. When treating a baby or an adult, I use my hands to envelop the wounded tissue and swaddle it like a baby wrapped up in a blanket. You want a snug fit but you don't want to press and push. In the same way water wraps around you in the Liquid Trust Fall, I ask my hands to encompass and support the inflamed tissue. Then, I listen, and feel for the intrinsic rhythm of the living cells within.

If your mind is unable to interpret an event, you will EmoThink about it in an attempt to process it. Your body is the battery that stores the voltage that fuels volatile EmoThoughts that inflame you. Your neural software informs your anatomical hardware in the same way computers implement code, just like how actors implement the script. Your body physically acts out your script, enacting crashed characters or healthy ones.

**Getting Into Character**

When actors play a role, they don't just say the lines, they feel the emotions and they embody their character's identity. Their neurochemistry is altered when they enact the trials and tribulations of their character, including success or failure, redemption or tragedy. Actors make the story real in their own body, and their genuine experience is contagious, because the audience also feels those feelings in their own bodies. Everyone's biochemistry is indelibly altered by their internal experiences, even though they were generated by a fictional, virtual scenario. Actors are the bridge that transforms an abstract script into a tangible experience in the audience. Who says dreams aren't real?

When you EmoThink, you're playing that character by reading their lines in your mind and actively feeling their emotions in your body. The more you believe you are this character, the more your biochemistry is altered as you say what they say and feel what they feel. Good actors win awards when they truly believe, and their belief makes them convincing. This phenomenon of believing in a story is called *suspension of disbelief*, where you agree to have a vicarious experience by empathizing with mythical characters. Even though you know it is a fictional story, you are willing to pretend it is real. When you "make believe", you take the quantum leap from pretending to believing, which changes your biochemistry and **makes it real.** Like the placebo effect, stories take advantage of the fact that we are highly suggestible. The Reboot also utilizes this fact and teaches you to hypnotize yourself into a highly relaxed state. Permission is one of my favorite words because it allows you to override your disbelief, surrender to the story, and induce a trance. Like Einstein's Thought Experiments, we can vet our dreams and see if they deserve our belief, but before we discount them, we must explore them and act them out, virtually and somatically.

### You Are An Ensemble Cast

You are a pantheon of personas, an array of archetypes, a constellation of characters. The stenographer names and identifies the various voices rumbling around inside your head, which means that you are not just a solo performer, you are an ensemble cast. You are a hodgepodge of many distinct impulses. If you consider that the amygdala in your brain is an adrenal watchdog and your limbic system wants to bond, you can see how you have both systems operating at the same time, all the time. Your brain's executive function is the "you" that has some influence over whether you are sympathetic or parasympathetic, friendly or foe-minded. Permission empowers your executive puppeteer to override the adrenal imperative, so you can play a healthier character. When you fully embody this version of you, your healthy self assumes the lead role and becomes the star. Your biochemistry follows, as it always does. The reactive, sickly character you used to identify with is now getting reimagined. I ask you to be versatile and capable of playing different characters, rather than always being typecast in similar roles. If it seems overwhelming to wear so many hats, you've already been practicing.

I introduced the Trust Falls of Relaxation by saying puppets enact scenes from stories. I asked you to become Raggedy Ann, and pretend that you are entirely passive and limp. It feels amazing! Thinking about being relaxed is a start, but you don't convince anyone until you Feel it in your body. Our Italian stick puppet is a different character, who adds the seed of desire, with a recurrent dream of becoming a human child. This vision to be autonomous replaces the puppeteer's hand above with a nervous system and free will. To really nail this role and win an award you'll need to Feel what it's like to have your body moved by mysterious strings that you have no control over. Pino also hears words come out of his mouth, even though he is not involved in choosing the words. He doesn't even have lungs that empower his voice. Everything he says and does is dictated. The only place he has any control is in his imagination, so he dreams of being his own puppeteer. He can't manifest his vision with his puppet body, so he dreams of upgrading it. He unplugs his old self and awakens Rebooted.

For us humans, the puppeteer is sitting at the dimmer console. Turning up a dimmer pulls a string and shortens a muscle. Because thoughts turn up dimmers, your bones are being pulled by your subliminal self-talk and your emotions. The part of you that EmoThinks is the part that is told what to say, how to feel, and what to do. There's no free will or conscious choice involved. So, for you to play Pino and get into this persona, recognize that you yourself are beholden to the neural software that generates EmoThoughts and stress. Recognize how powerful your programming is, trapping you in your personality. Even if you get frustrated and you throw a tantrum, you're still just reacting to your programming. How can you escape this prison that dictates your thoughts and emotions? You'll find the essence of this character in the longing to be free. Ask Buddha for help!

The Slow-Motion Trust Fall gives you the ability to watch yourself falling in slow motion, which gives you enough time to safely feel what's happening. Find your stride and settle into your own rhythm. The Liquid Trust Fall asks you to let go of Pino's orthopedic body and sink into your cells. This role is a radical departure from the humanoid puppets like Raggedy and Pino because this character is a jellyfish. To get here, you have to let go of your familiar human form of sticks and strings. In a weird way, this liberates your stick-puppet self and reimagines an entirely different body. While it might not seem more evolved than the mechanical you, if you feel the vibrations through your liquid body, you venture beyond the limiting programs that cause your neural software to crash. Working with this vibration improves how the glial cells in your brain function, which helps your neurons run advanced operations while staying cool. In contrast, EmoThinking and neural static create a shrill vibration of cognitive dissonance, overheating the brain and drying it out. Like whale songs permeating the vast ocean, harmonic brain waves create resonant overtones that exude wisdom. Thinking makes you smart, while wisdom is a fluid state of being. This series culminates with Free Fall, where you unplug your motor system with the master dimmer. Full permission is radical Release. When you shed all excuses, and commit to Release, you dive chest first into the open sky. Let it all go and toss yourself into the unknown.

Early in my career, many doctors remarked that acupuncture only worked if you believe in it. I had treated my roommate's dog, and the results were obvious. I refuted the idea that it was just a placebo because I don't think the dog had any concept or belief about acupuncture. I invited any skeptic to receive 2 treatments and then judge for themself if it helped. I often said that **my medicine is stronger than your doubt**. Most people felt improvement and were "won over" after they experienced a tangible benefit. A story must be compelling to earn the right to suspend disbelief, so my medicine must meet this standard to get through to a skeptic, or a dog that has no preconceptions. If a story rings true, it's easier for the audience to recognize the value of the tale. Actors actively believe they are their character, so they Feel deeply. The more you Feel, the more medicinal your meditations become.

**Contests Test Contestants**

Stories hinge on the protagonist being tested, and illness is the ultimate challenge. When the chips are down, we discover what we're made of. Today I attended a memorial service for a remarkable patient who was steadfast and graceful, despite serious physical impairment and chronic pain. I can only hope to be so eloquent as I live out my TimeLine, and enact Adrian's personal narrative!

Stories set up a plot that puts our character in a corner and confronts them with an essential choice that exposes their deepest nature. Their beliefs get challenged as they respond to their conditions, and we get to learn from their experiences as we vicariously live through them. Sporting events, chess matches, and card games set up a drama where two or more players Fight, so spectators can feel the thrill of victory or the agony of defeat. Contests and stories represent the real-world imperative to survive, the crucible that determines who lives and who dies. The pressure to survive sets the stage for all of the trials and tribulations of every living thing. Each and every organism is acting out their uniquely personal story, and we are all doing it in real time. Sports and stories are a safe training ground to practice how we handle threats, so we can sharpen our skills to convert traumas into lessons, improving our chances of survival. Even virtual battles are deeply consequential because every cell is working hard to help you win. When your team wins the big game, your exaltation is real.

External forces always act on you, and your circumstances shape your experience of things. Yet your response to your conditions generates your own internal forces that compel you to act in the ways you do. Free will allows you to decide and choose, rather than just react reflexively and robotically. I could write a whole book about external forces and the circumstances of our natural world, but I'd rather talk about you! Let's investigate the forces you generate from within. The Reboot gives you permission to go inside and Accept Feel Release each experience, to let them pass through you cleanly. These events don't define you, they refine you. Like raw steel gets heated and pounded by a blacksmith into a tool, nature forges characters who seek to survive. Actions speak louder than words, so let's distinguish reactions from your genuine will. **The Stenographer is willing to see and the Actor is willing to believe.** The question before you now is: what are your core beliefs?

## BelieveMoThoughts

By now you have habituated to the idea of EmoThoughts, so I'll add belief to the equation. In the Intrinsic Breath chapter, I described how the adrenal mind uses thinking to decide whether to Freeze Flight Fight and emotions add the motivation that executes the decree to play dead, run away, or attack. In physics, forces are vectors, which have a magnitude and a direction. We draw vectors as arrows that have a length (the energy behind it) and a direction (where the energy is focused). Emotion is the eMotive force that propels the arrow and thoughts direct your emotional energy toward the target. Your EmoThoughts dictate your behavior, which is what you actually do in the world.

We can say there are two types of actions, internal biochemical actions and external dimmer decisions. Lifting your arm in the air happens when you turn up a dimmer, shorten a muscle, and apply a force to your bone to overpower gravity and move. Internally, when you feel happy or sad, you secrete neurotransmitters and hormones that cause chemical reactions to occur within your cells. EmoThoughts turn up dimmers and they also cause chemical reactions, which amount to your inner and outer behavior. While sitting still and watching a horror movie, you are apparently not doing anything, but your muscles are tight and your cells are acting out Freeze mode. Even when you are asleep, you are acting out your programming. The only question is: which programs you are running?

We all gravitate toward our deeper beliefs, even if you think the placebo effect is hogwash. Religious zealots and ardent atheists are both convinced with absolute belief, so their fervor has them trapped. I've got a sharp acupuncture needle poised to pop your bubble of beliefs that inspire the EmoThoughts that compel your behavior. We're going to challenge our beliefs so that we can reprogram our EmoThoughts and change our biochemical behavior.

**Beliefs are the base layer of your operating system, your default settings.** Beliefs set up the programs that you follow. If you believe you're worthless, you'll run that program and fulfill that assumption. Our teenage driver feels unsafe while the car is moving, so they panic and cause an accident. When they relax behind the wheel, they implement a safer program, one that doesn't crash. Their inner safety is translated through their behavior, and they become a safe driver. Once you believe something, whatever it is, you invest in the entire belief system. You're not just merging with that one belief, you're connecting to all of the implications of that belief. This attaches you to an entire *belief system*. Once you *identify* with it, it becomes part of you. Now that you're invested, you "care", and you generate emotional energy to support your beliefs. The trouble with latching onto beliefs is that you quickly lose touch with reality. If you believe someone wants to harm you, you'll be compelled to strike first in preemptive self-defense. You become the perpetrator, even if you are wrong. In this case, your adrenal mind goes into Fight mode, generating thoughts that justify your behavior, claiming your attack is in self-defense.

When you merge yourself with an abstract belief system, if someone attacks these beliefs, they attack you. Before you know it, you're defending your beliefs. Your emotions mobilize your adrenal mind to think up arguments to defend your beliefs and justify your worldview. This need to be right makes people do outrageous things and it increases suffering within you and outside of you. You'll also want to discredit any viewpoints that contradict your perspective, so you'll pick them apart (Fight) or ignore them (Freeze). When other paradigms are radically different from your own, they challenge your assumptions. When threatened, your adrenals chime in, and your vagus nerve misfires. Now your investment in your beliefs has you falling into Freeze Flight Fight. This isn't a trust fall; you're just tripping.

Old beliefs are obsolete and need an update. Relativity and quantum mechanics pose a threat to classical thinking, our antiquated and oversimplified concept of spacetime. Buddhism recognizes that any beliefs lock you in a crashed loop of illusion, which causes suffering. Bruce Lee's central method was to not have a method. Instead of dogma, meet the moment directly. Your assumptions slow you down, and when they don't sync up with reality, you've got a blind spot. You don't need EmoThoughts to function and you don't need to identify with any beliefs either. They are just a security blanket that you carry around to feel safe, so when you are safe in your body, you can untether yourself and be free.

I proposed that Flight is the opposite of Feel, which I represent as a protective **shield in front of your heart**. Rigidly investing in your beliefs hardens the shield and keeps your heart locked up. You can't radiate love or wisdom if you're busy defending beliefs. When I introduced the 3 Principles, I said Feeling helps you define what this $x$ is. After you Accept that $x=x$, you can really look at the exact value of this experience, the absolute value. Beliefs skew your vision and blur the intrinsic truth of whatever reality is, like looking in a fun-house mirror. Once you Accept the fact that reality is unfathomable, you can stop trying to make sense of everything and you can flow with what is. If you want to be healthy, stop fighting the world, and join the HereNow!

Rather than holding on to what you think you know, I invite you to deconstruct your beliefs and live without them. As soon as you believe in something, you embody that character and you act out their lines, their program. Actors rely on the power of belief and stories utilize the placebo effect to influence your body and mind. I recommend the anti-placebo of *blank belief*. You've got to be passionate about being dispassionate, and believe in non-belief. Like judgments, beliefs generate suffering. Your need to be right and redeem yourself traps you in debilitating crashed loops.

## Be The Star Of Your Inner Show

The Stenographer produces the script. Now that you have your script written down, and you have identified the various characters that are speaking in your head, you can enact the scene. Your Reboot Camp Drill Sergeant is now your acting coach who helps you get into character and become the EmoThinking voices you are generating.

If you relate to being the Defendant who is accused of some flaw, you might have a harder time playing the harsh Prosecutor. Recently, while working with a young woman who was molested by her father and still traumatized by it, I asked her to consider that she had adopted this harsh voice that relentlessly shames her. Even though she learned about disempowerment from the outside, she internalized these lessons, and she is the one continuing to subliminally abuse herself. She is a kind person who wouldn't hurt a fly, yet in her own mind, she is vicious. Her Inner Perpetrator knows all her secrets and weaponizes everything against her. It took a while for her to wrap her head around this idea that she is also the Perpetrator, but then she got a handle on that voice that harms her.

The next step is to truly own this character by playing them convincingly. Really feel the vitriol and rancor they feel as they attack and try to hurt the *other*. That voice might be enraged, devoid of morals, or criminally insane. While it seems dangerous to become this character, it is more dangerous to try and bury this voice and lock it up in solitary confinement. This character won't just evaporate or disappear, it will continue to EmoThink and seep into your body, causing dysfunction. Anything unprocessed stays in the system! It gets stored in your subconscious mind and your somatic body, causing mental and cellular stress.

For this reason, enacting these voices is a sound strategy. It's a delicate undertaking: daring to Feel the emotions of the vicious perpetrator or a worthless victim. However, if we don't Accept and Feel, we can't Release. Once you tap into the hate that fuels these voices, you can let go of them and transform these personas. Like an antidote neutralizes poison by converting toxins into harmless molecules, Accept Feel Release transmutes imbalanced energy into neutral Qi. If you dare to Feel, please apply the 3rd Principle of Release, and let go of whatever you experienced. This keeps you safe from getting lost in the dark places that can be overwhelming. The Reboot is the gift that keeps on giving....

# Release: Write a New Story

Now that you know your script and you have acted out your various characters, you can approach the task of letting go of this old narrative. To take this final step, you are no longer the actor who embodies the familiar characters. Become the writer who dreams up new characters, and imagine your best self. To really capture this healthier persona, you need to cleanse any residue from the tragic versions you have been playing for years. This takes you even deeper into the false beliefs and reactive motivations that caused the old character's hardship. To cultivate this new you, surrender the self that suffered. Letting go of the part of you that was wounded sows seeds in your imagination, which envisions a better way that bears fruit. To liberate your enlightened persona and allow it to shine, fully Release what was and master the Fight response. Earlier I mentioned false detachment as a shortcut that skips ahead to Release. It doesn't work that way because you can't let go of something you don't have: you have to attach before you detach. *Trying* to let go is just forcing it, which is actually Fight mode, not flow. Forgiveness 2.0 weaves forgiveness with the 3 Principles, so you can complete the process and awaken. Claim authority and grant yourself permission to decommission the old you, and unplug the familiar characters you previously embodied.

This chapter explores the transition from Flight to Fight, which delves into the complex interaction between the victim mentality and the willingness to perpetrate against an *other*. Abused people have a keen understanding of how it feels to be wounded, so they are educated in how to inflict similar wounds on those weaker than them. Sometimes rather than fighting the stronger bully, people find someone weaker to pick on. When a victim is ready to step out of Flight mode, they will often get pulled toward the Fight response, which sets up the pecking order. In this dog-eat-dog world, the cycle of abuse keeps going because hurt people, hurt people. Victims who are trained in abuse often become the best perpetrators. This cause-and-effect relationship stirs the karmic loop where an abused victim becomes an abusive perpetrator, who then creates another abused victim, who then eventually fights back, etc. This chapter also illustrates how quantum entanglement offers lessons in resolving the oppositional forces of yin/yang. Fortunately, Release breaks this vicious cycle and liberates us from reacting, which elevates our consciousness.

When I introduced the 3 Principles, I said they are in a natural order, and the 3F's of Freeze Flight Fight are the mirror image of disorder. Attempting to claim power by disempowering others sets up the pecking order, and nature demonstrates that survival of the fittest favors this strategy. Aggression is advantageous because the impulse to use your energy, resources, and will against your opponent improves your chances of survival. Although I have been railing against the adrenals for 200 pages, nature clearly prefers this strategy, at least in the short-term. I'm contending that long-term survival relies on converting the Fight response into Release. Freeze is the inability to Accept and Flight is an unwillingness to Feel. War is the opposite of peace, and peace is the key to Release.

On page 86 I introduced the concept of Personal Power, which is an adrenal ladder toward safety. Now I'll flesh out this idea with a simple equation: safety = control. The adrenals want to get safe, and getting safe means having control over your environment, so you have a safe space. If you had control over everything, you could neutralize any threat. Freezing concedes all space, including the space within your physical body. Freeze is traumatic because you dissociate and leave your body, so you don't belong anywhere. Flight seeks to move your body away from the threat, so you concede the external space around your body and seek another safe space to occupy. Even though Fight is hurtful and opens the door to abuse, it is progress because you push back on the external assault and you try to reclaim your outer environment. Sometimes, offense is the best defense.

The impulse to Fight is a good thing, if we remain careful to direct our anger wisely. Otherwise, we oversteer like a teenage driver and we recklessly crash, hurting others and creating more victims. All victims need to reclaim their power at some point, which inspires them to fight back and attack those who injured them. Before long we all trade wounds. The adage "power corrupts, and absolute power corrupts absolutely" describes how the Fight response corrupts power by wielding it to harm another. In the context of the pecking order, weaponized power and aggression are rewarded, but raw aggression fails the test of creating anything. If you want a new character to play, you need to channel their aggression in a creative way. Otherwise, you'll just write another revenge story about grievance and karmic pay back. If our lead character works through their trauma and lets bygones be bygones, they pay it forward. The story is uplifting, rather than depicting tragic ends.

## The Pendulum Of Passive Aggression

The passive-aggressive interplay is everywhere in relationships among family, friends, and rivals. If someone either neglects you or lashes out at you, your feelings get hurt. Until you forgive them unconditionally, you'll EmoThink about it and you'll go through the phases of Freeze Flight Fight. Your behavior reflects your emotions, so you will be closed, distant, or rude. Depending on your mood and the situation, you might bounce back and forth between feeling shamefully weak or aggressive. As you react to your adrenal mind, you oscillate between the passive victim and the vindictive perpetrator, transitioning from Flight to Fight and back again. Forgiveness breaks the cycle because you Feel the hurt and then Release it. When you are no longer injured, you don't need to push back against the insult. You can see it for what it is, and eventually arrive at forgiveness. Forgiveness emanates from a healed place because you are no longer wounded, in the sense that you don't identify as a victim. You might have scars, but now you are safe, and your adrenals aren't necessary. Now you can Accept Feel Release instead, so you can be your best self that is present and parasympathetic. If you are still hurting, your EmoThoughts compel you to churn and grind your way through the phases of Freeze Flight Fight. To navigate this challenge, redirect your impulse to attack. We can look to martial arts for guidance on how to use our power. Many disciplines teach students to be humble and to channel their aggressive energy in creative ways, while simultaneously building the skillset of a warrior. You also learn how to take a punch and get hurt, so part of the training is to Accept pain and tolerate it as a precondition.

Burying the problem (Freeze) or avoiding it (Flight) is not the answer. The trick is to confront the truth without anger. Fierce honesty works, because you are powerful and unafraid to face whatever is there. This is a healthy Fight response. You are willing to Feel everything, including pain. This deep Acceptance recognizes that this moment might hurt, yet you Accept it anyway. You refuse to Freeze because you are a **Sensory Warrior**, highly disciplined and willing to Feel what is. True to your training, you now apply Release and let go of that difficult moment. The obstacle course here is to conquer the myth that your experiences define you. Spoiler alert: they don't. Even if something hurt you and you suffered, your wounds do not encapsulate the entirety of you. When you Release them, they pass through you. We say "You are what you eat," but whatever you defecated is no longer you. It was temporarily housed in you GI tract, but when you excreted it, you detached from it. You extracted some nutrients from the food and internalized those, but you rejected most of the molecules. The analogy is to take the lesson from what happened, and leave the residue behind. The more cleanly you process molecules and moments, the healthier you are.

If you carry your past injuries into the present moment you're in, you are a victim of life. Your leg might be broken, and you might have scars, but that doesn't make you a victim. You become a victim when you identify with your wound and you use that to define yourself. I have worked with many hospice patients who were dying, yet they were not victims of their demise. They were tough enough to Accept what was happening, even though they wanted to live. If you are a Sensory Warrior, you Accept and Feel whatever cards you are dealt. Rather than playing the victim card, you work to become the wild card that redeems your hand. The Sensory Warrior creates safety and reclaims space by fiercely looking the unknown in the eye and standing strong with an open heart. You don't need to retreat and hide behind your shield. You also drop your sword because you refuse to attack as a means to protect yourself. This is the pinnacle of power, combining fierce fearlessness with compassionate kindness. It might seem like a strange combination at first, but try it out and see if it fits. Ferocity is fiery, but when you tame your inner flame, you channel your power toward the greater good. The trick is to disavow the victim persona while also disavowing the perpetrator. To shed your victim, you need to pick up a weapon and fight back. As soon as you match the aggression coming at you, drop your sword and soften. This subtle balance is how you convert the Fight impulse into Release, which unleashes your parasympathetic power.

Sensory Warriors are safe in their own skin. They have full command of their body and their mind can't be co-opted by adrenal fear. Accept Feel Release converts reactive anger into fierce friendship and potent presence. Your Sensory Warrior is not only in control; it is in command. You've got a budding new character emerging, and your Sensory Warrior is on track to becoming a leader, and the star of your new show. It's funny that people who are *controlling* are stressed and anxious, so they are not in command of their EmoThoughts or their dimmer switches. Fear makes teenage drivers dangerous. When they are justifiably confident, they make the outer world a safer place. When you conquer your adrenal mind and claim full authority over your Ego, your body becomes a safe place, and you radiate soft power. Now you can mediate between the warring factions within you and find common ground. Reject reactive anger, and can express more creative aspects of yourself. Your tense fighter evolves into a wise sage who is powerful yet poetic, like Yoda. I periodically smile when I imagine my Inner Prosector adopting a hobby, like gardening or pottery. All of the energy wasted on litigating "who did what" gets repurposed, transmuting vicious loops into compassion cycles. Once you sort through your reactive anger, you can feed the flow, and surf the Tao.

## Anger Is Pressure

If you overuse Freeze and Flight, you'll accumulate pressure and eventually pop a gasket. Enraged people explode and frustrated people vent, letting off steam. These phrases describe how anger relates to pressure. When you own your anger and truly claim your Inner Perpetrator, you realize that if someone triggers you, you are a loaded gun. If someone pushes your buttons, you're a bomb. The ammunition is yours, so blaming the other person for provoking you doesn't justify the pressure within you. Accept the fact that you are provokable, and your pent-up energy is your responsibility. There is no excuse for bad drivers who cut you off on the freeway, but your road rage is yours. Don't be so eager to cast the first stone, lest ye be judged. In fact, throwing a stone at someone shows that you are hazardous and a big part of the problem.

The reason you store all of this energy in your body's battery is because you identified as a victim. The weaker you felt, the more desperate you are to reclaim power, and the more explosive you become. When attacked, energy is projected at you. You might block some of it, but shields aren't strong enough to buffer all of it. Some energy gets absorbed and stored, increasing internal pressure. Each time you get insulted, you accumulate ammunition. Counterattacks use that pent up pressure, so **before you can own your anger, you need to own your inner victim.**

Picture two balloons that are touching and pressed together a bit, so there is a flat part where they indent each other. If they are inflated equally, the border is in the middle between the two balloons. If 25% of the air was taken out of one balloon, the boundary would shift toward the small balloon. If extra air were added to the full balloon, it would get bigger and encroach even more on the small balloon. Now imagine your personal space around you as a 3-foot balloon or bubble encircling your body. If you get angry, your balloon inflates. If you get attacked often, you might learn how to shrink up your balloon to minimize the violence of the attack. If you concede too much space, your balloon will get pressed all the way down to your skin. If your pressure drops even more, and your balloon is smaller than your body, the other person's balloon will enter your body and infiltrate your anatomy. This is when Freeze occurs, when the body's physical space is co-opted. If the balloon is smaller than you are, your defenses have been overridden and you conceded your somatic territory. If you inflate your balloon so that it is bigger than your skin, you are no longer frozen. Hooray!! If you keep inflating your personal bubble and push back toward the overinflated balloon, you'll claim more and more space. When you match the other person's pressure, you establish your personal domain and you occupy your rightful space.

It's interesting to see interactions in terms of these pressure bubbles. Study how inflated you are relative to the people around you in your daily life. Use your somatic skills to feel their pressure status. Fight is over-inflated, Flight is under-inflated, and Freeze is totally deflated. I see Freeze all the time in my patients' bodies, especially in the chest and throat. When I put my hands on traumatized tissue, it's as if the bubble caved in and got adhered to their anatomy. That part of the balloon's membrane cemented into the tissue, so their bubble was pinned down and unable to expand. The treatment frees the tissue, which liberates the bubble and allows it to inflate. The person occupies their neutral space, which is a huge relief, like taking off a tight wetsuit and taking a full breath.

Fighters are also locked up in their tissue. They emphatically resist imploding, so they attempt to generate pressure by squeezing down on their core. This backfires and implodes them even more than caving in. They end up hating their obstacles, which makes them less likely to transcend the challenge. Like straining to have a bowel movement, they try to push through the blockage. Often the extra pressure just makes it worse by hardening the wound that constricts them. If you have a complex knot in a string and you pull on it because you are frustrated, you just make it harder to untangle. When confronted with a knot, summon your Sensory Warrior and patiently address the restriction by applying the Principles.

**Chronic Cycles of Internal Abuse**

Most self-talk is an abusive relationship between the accuser and the accused. We can use the lens of Flight/Fight to better understand the dynamic between our victimized parts and our vindictive side. A typical domestic abuse scenario has the abuser getting enraged for whatever reason and beating up the vulnerable victim. After the outburst, the abuser might have remorse and promise to never do it again. Of course, this isn't the last time this happens, and once the pressure builds up again, the abuser shifts from remorse to rage. Low blood sugar, alcohol, and hormonal swings are just a few biological factors that influence the chronic anger that inflame ragaholics.

Why do the victims stay? The answer is embedded in the question: because they identify as a victim. If they were not a victim, they wouldn't stay. When animals are sufficiently cornered, they will do anything to get free, including risking their life. They realize that Freeze and Flight are inadequate, so they adopt Fight. An addict hits rock bottom when they exhaust their drug, and victims hit rock bottom when they exhaust avoidance. They can't hide or deflect their way out of this predicament, so they finally face it head on. Accepting chronic abuse is what makes a victim a victim. If we look at how people habituate and grow accustomed to harsh things like smoking cigarettes, we see how the fear of change keeps people stuck in a suboptimal status quo. Our ability to adapt makes us amazingly tolerant, sometimes to a fault. When a victim finally sheds their Frozen or Flighty persona, they Fight back. When cornered, they're willing to risk everything to refuse the abuse. When victims tap their raw survival impulse, all of their stored adrenaline gets expressed as an attack. This inflates their balloon and redraws the boundary. It's a necessary step in the right direction, but it doesn't really pan out in the long run, because all adrenal defenses only offer a temporary fix. Like Freeze and Flight, Fight is just a passing phase.

Can you recall an occasion when you were particularly mean to yourself? During the remorse phase, when your angry side realized they were out of control, the victim can point the finger and accuse the abusive voice of foul play. However justified they may be, the victim might also be angry about being berated, so they might vilify the abuser and seek to punish them. The abused part might have disdain and vitriol for the abuser who is suddenly sorry. Now, the victim is righteously lashing out at the abuser, which makes them a perpetrator. It seems fair but it doesn't resolve the relationship. The abuser becomes a victim, and the victim is now willing to avenge their wound. In an effort to regain power, victims transition from Flight to Fight, which sets up their next attack. When we oscillate between abuser and abused, we enact the pecking order in our own BodyMind, and we suffer the collateral damage.

The problem with regret and shame is that they don't teach you anything or help you atone for your transgressions. The abuser must **perform and act of service** to regain integrity. The next time you notice a critical tone in your head, shift your righteous indignation to how a kindergarten teacher works with a stubborn kid. Rather than yell and scream to coercive them to obey, good teachers focus their voice and speak directly to the child who is stuck in a funk. They exert the soft power of the judge who doesn't judge, the parent who is safe, yet strong. The kid is not going to get away with anything because they are being confronted with their own behavior. Also, the child is not being shamed and belittled for messing up, because they are shown a path to restoring integrity. If they take the off-ramp and see the error of their ways, they have a chance to change. We all lose our way sometimes, and we can be forgiven. If we learn this lesson and amend our behavior, we might even earn the right to be trustworthy in the future. Instead of the dominant adult crushing the child's bubble, the teacher helps the kid self-regulate and find their neutral space, which isn't aggressive or brooding. Everyone involved actually becomes empowered from this process, rather than getting swallowed by the vicious cycle of negative reinforcement. As with the trust falls, the more you trust, the easier it gets, so you can jump from a higher perch.

Beyond the intrapersonal politics of who's right or wrong, if you have a harsh voice in your head, you are being verbally abused. This subliminal abuse means that part of you is actively suffering in this moment. You can sweep it under the rug and pretend you're fine, but you'll get a stiff upper lip and your face will freeze a bit. The wound remains. Criticism is a mild micro-aggression cloaked under the guise of teaching and accountability. "I should have done that better," etc. conflates the assessment of a better way with the judgment of *should*. Another common phrase you might say to yourself is "That was a dumb thing to do," which is a bit harsher. Other self-talk that include words like "bad" are outright hostile, so they qualify as macro-aggressions. In contrast to an obviously violent beheading in one swift stroke, the hen pecking of *should* is death by a thousand cuts. Either way, **stress is abuse**, and abuse is a misuse of power.

Actors demonstrate how EmoThoughts create biochemical changes, which have real world consequences for your human body. Self reproach weakens you on every level, plain and simple. To whatever degree, the beliefs that fuel your judgments are willing to harm an innocent animal on the planet. We're all just trying to survive. Your human body is an amazing feat of evolution, and although it is highly imperfect, it is sacred and beautiful. Because the body enacts and embodies the mind, psychological abuse becomes physical suffering. Turning up dimmers shortens the muscles running parallel to your spine, compressing discs, causing back and neck pain. When your vagus nerve backfires, your gut goes berserk. Background tension makes your breathing shallow. Is this ok with you? Would you kick a dog because you had a bad day? I doubt it, yet if you berate any living being, including yourself, for any reason, you are an abuser who is violating the rights of a creature of nature, a proverbial child of God. Every living being is imbued with the inalienable right to life, liberty, and pursuit of nirvana … not just transient happiness! **I often feel like an animal rights activist, protecting my patients' body from their mind**. I beg them to be kind to themselves, or at least less harsh. To find this deep peace and arrive at Release, you must Accept and Feel what is, even if it's ugly.

## The Corset And The Collar:  A Grim Fairy Tale

I defined the Intrinsic Breath as the body in its natural state, breathing in and out all by itself. The goal is to get out of the way of the breath, witness the body breathe, and acknowledge that the body is breathing. Getting out of the way means that we are not involved, we are the witness. As I was exploring this ability to witness, I pictured a naturalist observing animals in their natural state. If the scientist were to make noise, become known, and be recognized by the animals, then this would disturb the natural state. The animals would react to this outsider, changing the dynamic by imposing an interaction. Rather than a true observation of the animals in their natural state, the clumsy naturalist can only register their response. So often, when we become aware of our breath, we judge it reflexively and therefore we are interacting with it right away. We rarely get an opportunity to just witness the body breathe, because we are so quick to jump in there and try to fix it or make it better. To be a witness, you have to sneak up and stalk your Intrinsic Breath in the same way a naturalist must remain invisible to just be an observer. This vital skill enables you to actually learn something about yourself by witnessing your physiology, rather than jumping in and trying to fix it in a crude way. Quieting the judgmental voices makes your presence invisible, so you don't disturb your natural state.

I continued to ponder our relationship to animals. We often either tame animals by feeding them and coercing them kindness, or we subjugate them with repressive methods and straight-up domination. A choke collar is a device that constricts the throat, which is a very effective way to get an animal's attention and to communicate to that animal that you command their life 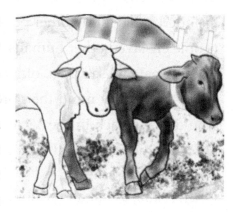 force. Pulling on the leash not only directs their attention and moves them, squeezing the collar chokes them. This restricts their ability to breathe, and asserts dominion over their life. When you digest this harsh truth, you realize a choke collar is a horrible device.

A cage confines an animal in a box, like a prison cell, whereas a corset is a cage that you wear. Depending on the size of the cage, you might be able to pace around, whereas a corset is an overtly physical cage, in the sense that it is on the body. A tight corset binds the movement of the torso and therefore restricts breathing. Like a collar around the throat, a corset constrains the body and compromises the breath. It's staggering to recognize the negativity of these common devices we invented that brutalize animals and ourselves. Being accountable for our behavior requires deep humility because to fully comprehend what we have done

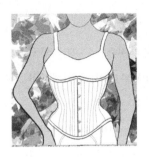

demands that we Feel the wounds we inflicted on living beings. Accountability leads to atonement, and forgiving those responsible for causing harm. This doesn't excuse any transgressions; it simply ends the endless cycle of wounding.

The next phase of my Thought Experiment invoked the British Empire, which dominated the world for several centuries by colonizing other lands, usurping natural resources, and harnessing the wildlife. Colonization also included subjugating other peoples, so humans didn't just enslave animals, people enslaved other humans. Race, gender, and class are among the ways we delineate these strata, of who is subjugated and who is not, like a cruel caste system. My mind then presented me with images of how the British would dress back in the Victorian times. The corset was a device women used and men often had tight collars. It seems odd, but a necktie is a leash.

I then realized that all the abuse imperialists wrought on their colonies was not personal, it was spilling out from inside of them and onto others. In the book *The 4 Agreements*, the first Agreement is: nothing is personal. Because BelievEmoThoughts lead to behavior, our actions are the result of our internal condition, so when we injure others, we just acting out what is inside of us. The Brits didn't just repress others, they subjugated their own animal nature. Their attitude that animals are property was also how they viewed their own bodies, so they repressed themselves too. This doesn't excuse their atrocities, it merely frames what happened, that we might understand our common history. When we look at perpetrators who dominate other creatures, whether they are animals or people, ultimately the perpetration is internal. That voice inside their head that pushes them to dominate and disempower another is in their head. The perpetration is inside of them and spilling out into the outside world, so they are expressing their subliminal script and acting out their inner story.

This gets to the crux of clearing ourself and discharging any lingering charges of being a victim. Forgiveness is so fundamental because we must fully acknowledge our own Inner Perpetrator inside of us. If you don't suppress yourself, you won't be eager to repress people, animals, or the planet. If you feel weak, you'll seek power over *other*. Stress is an excuse to keep spinning the karmic wheel of suffering and the vicious cycle of discord. A perpetrator injures the victim and bad karma is vaguely associated with getting hurt or bad luck. Karmic justice is the flip side, where the victim regains some power when the perpetrator gets wounded. Ideally, they can now commiserate because they have a shared, common injury. If they both learned a lesson, they won't need to repeat trading wounds with adrenal overreactions. The crudest way to get power is to hurt someone else and put them below you. The pecking order is a survival spectrum. If you get beat down by someone, you can beat someone else down and be somewhere in the middle, and not at the bottom. Our survival depends on working to get ourselves up this ladder, which is a very slippery karmic ladder. The problem is you can't actually evolve and escape the maze of the adrenal mind from this process. Tragically, this is why suffering is endemic and perpetuated over generations.

If we are to change the narrative here, we must acknowledge the complex role that we have as victim and perpetrator. Professor Zero says: "When you think a thought, you turn up a dimmer." Often, the dimmers you turn up constrict your breath. If you create tension in your torso, then you're creating a corset. If there's any tension in your throat. you are tightening your choke collar. Your nervous system is certainly aware of the narrowing of the tube, so there is an awareness within your cellular self of construction in the throat, which is a compromise in your airway, which is distressing. When an animal gets their collar squeezed, they perk up, become attentive, and obey. When your mind is running amok and thinking, especially shameful and self-deprecating thoughts, then the body, your body, is actually being abused. This is a very precarious situation for the body to be in. When the throat and torso are tight, your body is being punished for no good reason. Anxiety tightens the noose and restricts your actual LifeForce.

I judge that this is wrong. The body does not deserve to be treated in this way. The body is not responsible for those thoughts, because it didn't create the problems or the shame that you feel. The body then becomes objectified, and is subjected to those feelings that you have. If you acknowledge and take ownership of your perpetration over your own body, in the sense of stress creating the corset and the collar that constricts your ability to breathe, then you have a chance to stop doing this. This is a liberation opportunity to stop self-subjugation. Shame is driving all of the perpetration that we witness because the perpetrators are reacting to their victimhood by acting out their toxic concept of self. If you have self-esteem, you will recognize that every living being also has rights. You will bow to them with respect, honor their path through life, and even support them. Vilifying your fellow villagers, even if they are totally wrong, poisons the well from which we all drink. Acting out doesn't just hurt you, it is the choice to weaponize and inflict harm.

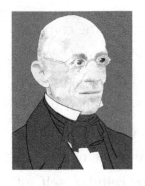

The breathing-balloon imagery from the Reboot meditation is your ticket to freedom. I ask you to relax your tongue and open the tube, which removes your collar and liberates your airway. When you feel the back of the balloon massaging the kidneys, you are unlacing your corset and allowing your lungs to fill and empty. After I delved into this Thought Experiment that became the Corset and the Collar fable, I realized it lined up perfectly with the Reboot Method that targets the throat (vagus) and the kidneys (adrenals). I smile at this symmetry, and I hope it helps you take this medicine into your body and actualize your healing. Please unshackle yourself from the yoke of needless tension, that you might find peace. To clarify my request, I'm not asking you to dream about some abstract idea of peace. I stand before you, inviting you to experience peace in your body, right HereNow. The Sensory Warrior's first act is to respond to constriction with compassion. Turning off your dimmers Releases your own suffering, and when you feel relief, your heart opens and you become benevolent. You see the value in being kind to your body, which is an innocent animal that is just trying to live. Once you salvage your self, you can serve by alleviating the suffering of others. Likewise, if you are shackled, your suffering leaks out and injures others.

The moral of this fable: Free yourself and radiate peace!
Internal vilification inevitably spills out and infects the outer world.

## Equal and Opposite Reactions: Introduction to yin/yang

Reboot Camp described habituation, which is how we adapt to things. I said adapting is a double-edged sword because when you adapt to smoking, you tolerate a suboptimal condition. Everyone with chronic stress has acclimated to their corset and their collar. Newton's 1st law of motion describes inertia, which says that a body's momentum will tend to remain constant unless acted upon by a force. Inertia is a natural phenomenon that describes how bodies resist changing their trajectory. Habituation is how behavior becomes ingrained as your not-so-new normal. Like computers running code, habits have mechanical, mindless momentum.

The Trust Falls of Relaxation invoke equilibrium by exploring how bodies in motion become bodies at rest. A falling body is acted upon by the force of gravity, which accelerates it toward the ground. Raggedy teaches us that when you're on solid ground, you have permission to turn off your dimmers. As a clinician, my job is to apply a force that alters the inertia of a diseased body, tilting it toward health. To generate this force capable of altering ingrained inertia, I guide patients to their center. Rebooting is sinking into your own personal equilibrium, and attaining homeostasis. When Raggedy Ann lies in stillness, the gravity that pulls her is matched by the ground that holds her, balancing the opposing forces. Catching yourself brings your wounded, fractured parts back to home base, to the caring heart beating in your chest.

Inertia says things are static and they don't change. Cycles repeat and maintain the status quo, like clockwork. Newton's 2nd law describes a force that influences the body and alters its inertia. Things change if and when a force is applied. In high school I was taught this was an "external force", but recent versions don't specify where the force comes from, so I'll focus on **forces that are generated internally**. Your life is a product of your cellular mitochondria, churning out the Qi that becomes the electricity that propels your heart and diaphragm. You were born with abundant will, but it might not be strong enough to alter your inertia unless you cultivate your awareness and ability through training. Do you remember being a Reboot Camper and being confronted with the obstacle course? This is where you found a crack on the wall that gave you a foothold. You also got a grip. When your energy and attention are focussed on your ground, however tenuous it might be, your will is expressed. You get a leg up to do what you intend to do and you accomplish something. If you slip and slide, your will doesn't create a practical result in the real world.

Newton's 2nd law describes **forces altering inertia**, which changes the trajectory of a body. You can hope and pray that an outside force will magically alter you condition, like wishing you get dealt a wild card. Your job to self-heal is to become your own wild card, and to produce an internal force. Don't sit around and expect the angels to save you, redeem yourself! Become your own joker! Do the work to attain SelfEmpathy, which fosters the force of compassion that can tip the scales toward your own good.

Newton's 3rd law of motion states: for every action there is an equal and opposite reaction, which describes a symmetrical relationship between static inertia and dynamic change. As an acupuncturist, I see oppositional forces as yin/yang, and I balance these forces within my patients. As an amateur mathematician, I relate *equal and opposite* to how every number has a negative counterpart, a mirror image, a quantumly entangled twin. As a physics enthusiast, I see how positive and negative charges attract and repel each other with equal force yet opposite direction. Like binary charge, spin is a fundamental, symmetrical property. When a vicious cycle spins in the other direction, it becomes a compassion cycle. Healing occurs when a diseased state is transmuted into its counterpart, a healthy state. Through a geometric lens, a body's mirror image is exactly the same as the original, only the left/right symmetry is inverted and reversed. *Equal yet opposite* is the common thread that links all of these truths. Newton's 3rd law describes the mechanical reality, electromagnetism accurately describes how opposing charges create valence and voltage, while yin/yang and mathematics describes the overall property of symmetry and duality.

## The Rebound: The Push/Pull of Flight and Fight

After being confined for a while, you might run as soon as you're sprung free. You might also lash out if you're cornered. This is the moment the rabbit runs for it or the cornered animal attacks. If we avert the Freeze response of mental implosion, we do something and we actively try to get safe. After you snap out of the trance of frozen EmoThinking, which is deliberating between Flight and Fight mode, you finally make a decision and you act. You either run away from the threat or toward it. You'll run at the same speed, but in the opposite direction because you are either attracted to or repelled by the situation. The parts of you that are frozen and dissociated are stunned and they don't have any choices. If you are recently unfrozen, you only have two choices, the binary dilemma of Fight

213

or Flight. With all of the adrenaline floating around in your bloodstream, you will implement your survival strategy of defense or offense. The remedy for the defensive reaction is to drop your shield, stand strong, and Feel. Release is the remedy for the Fight response.

## Drop Your Sword

To bury the hatchet and end the abuse, take a vow of non-violence. Get on your knees, lay your body down like Raggedy Ann, or look in the mirror: solemnly commit to not harming anyone, including yourself. Many have come before you and taken this oath and some have managed to successfully comply. Most of us are still working on it because we slip up and succumb to the Fight response. Your Inner Healer takes the Hippocratic oath: do no harm. In Ayurveda and yoga, it's called Ahimsa. Buddhists endeavor to alleviate the suffering of all sentient beings, while Quakers are pacifists, rejecting the impulse to cause harm.

I remarked that I often feel like an animal-rights activist who speaks up for the suffering of animals against undue hardship. When you advocate for something or someone, you defend them by appealing to the conscience of the abuser. How do we awaken the conscience within our own consciousness? First, the Stenographer must see and hear everything clearly. We Accept what is, even if it is painful or traumatic. Second, we embody each character, own their identities, and empathize with everyone's perspective. Third, we detach cleanly, we forgive, and we appreciate the absolute value of the experience. We need to complete all 3 phases to awaken our conscience that holds us accountable in a productive way. Atonement is difficult, but tough love is still love.

To walk a peaceful path, begin with your EmoThoughts. To reprogram adrenal self-talk, imagine placing an alternate program in your neural software that rings a bell in your brain, reminding you to stop judging yourself harshly. When I palpate a patient or use an acupuncture needle, I ask them to take another look at their problem, which reframes how they perceive their issue. My treatments also challenge BelievEmoThoughts, to clear any judgments that cloud their perception of themself. By dispersing the fog of neural static, the faller and catcher finally see each other, which sets up the Trust Fall of Self Healing.

When an addict seeks treatment to quit, I don't focus on their behavior, so I don't tell them to stop using. I work on their inner dialogue, so they understand why they are overusing. Often, when they relapse, they feel shame and hate themselves, and I don't want to play into this cyclical punishment by pressuring them not to use. They want to stop, since they came to see me, so I help their Stenographer see why they use and why they want to quit. Both motivations are in them, and when they get untangled, the person can make a more conscious choice. When difficult emotions pop up, I coach them to Accept Feel Release, rather than escape. Each time they show up in this way, they gain a modicum of self-esteem and they become more trustworthy. In time, they build their will and generate enough force to alter their inertia and transform their behavior. To break these habitual cycles that have amassed inertia, we all need to own our own energy. This next segment describes how to work with your unresolved, adrenal parts that are stuck in Freeze Flight Fight. To fulfill the oath of non-violence, we must also look at the micro-aggressions we perpetrate against our self and those around us, so we can see how our BelievEmoThoughts influence our behavior. I will describe common patterns in relationships with loved ones, but these dynamics also apply to your relationship with yourself, as the various personas within you work out their power struggle.

**Freeze:** Don't harm yourself. Shame injures your Inner Child.
**Flight:** Don't harm self by avoiding or shrinking. Commit.
**Fight:** Don't harm anyone. No blame. Forgive whoever you are mad at.

**Freeze** injures the self because the frozen part has relinquished all power and they have no ground, no safe space. Often, this ideology includes the belief that they deserve the abuse they received. They continue to throw themselves under the bus, which reinforces the trauma and keeps it front and center. PTSD is so horrible because the nervous system is perpetually overwhelmed, so there is no solace or reprieve.

Being frozen also injures others, since being self-absorbed reduces the capacity to love, leaving friends out in the cold. Frozen parts can't trust anyone, including the self, so this lack of self-esteem makes it impossible to have healthy relationships. Their boundaries were bulldozed and they're still broken. If you listen carefully to the tone of some people's voice, you can hear the parts that are slightly shrill. The chronic tightness in the chest doesn't supply enough breath to power the vocal mechanism. The part that imploded into shame lost its voice. Reclaiming your voice is critical in relationships, so you can speak your truth and dare to be seen and heard.

Finding your voice also empowers your healthier cast of characters, including your forgiving Judge and your Sensory Warrior. The Inner Protector also plays a major role for your frozen parts, because the traumatized part isn't strong enough yet to handle the world; they need a safe ally whose only mission is to protect them. While friends can help with this, it's not fair to expect someone to drop their needs in order to fulfill yours. In the short-term that's fine, but if you are stubbornly attached to being frozen, you become a burden and an obligation to your partner. Eventually they will need something that nourishes them. They might neglect you or push you away to regain their center, which can then reinforce your belief that you are unworthy. You can fix this by doing your own work, finding your Inner Protector, and building up your voice.

There is often a love-hate vibe in relationships because the frozen persona desperately wants contact, but love gets conflated with abuse. This persona also relies too heavily on the spouse to give them purpose, so insecurity dominates them and they constantly need to have their value affirmed. It's almost impossible for couples to help each other with their frozen parts because each person has to do their own internal work. You can love your frozen partner and support them, but they must heal their broken self-esteem. Your confidence in them only goes so far, because the voices of shame can crush even pure love. They dismiss it if they *believe* they are unworthy, so that belief must change if they are to be liberated. In the same way Humpty can't be fixed by all the king's men, no other person can heal you or change your core beliefs.

If you look at Freeze using the personal-space bubbles, their bubble is smaller than their skin. The loving partner's energy bubble permeates the body of the frozen one, which helps, but it's still not their own energy, so they don't occupy their own space. Until they inflate their own balloon, they rely on their partner to dispel the demons that haunt their subliminal subconscious. Their Inner Protector fixes holes in the balloon and repairs their boundaries, consolidating internal energy and pumping up their balloon. Once the bubble gets bigger than their skin, they are no longer frozen!

**Flight** injures the self because there is still doubt and lack of authority. It's not fully committed yet. To remedy Flight, Feel with commitment and become the Sensory Warrior that is willing to experience whatever comes in, including pain. No conditions or excuses. Drop the shield and find your backbone. Instead of using your foothold to run away, use your connection to the ground to stand firm and claim the space you are in. This is how you gain ground. The flighty persona has some space but not enough, so it is still encroached upon. It is easy to resent being kept down, and this angst feeds the Fight response. *Flighters* still need to push back against whoever is repressing them, so they might strategically lash out, but in passive-aggressive ways. Flighters are coy about their attacks, and they don't own their transgressions because they pretend they didn't do anything. They feel justified, but their lack of commitment keeps them from really owning their aggression like fighters do.

If we look at the dynamics of personal-space bubbles, the challenge is to inflate yourself without attacking or hating the other person's overinflated balloon. Sometimes they are not really over-inflated; sometimes the problem is that you are under-inflated. If you inflate your bubble, the other person might accommodate, finding a happy medium. Other times they are a true enemy, and you need to dig deep to muster the will to make a stand. Are you committed to claiming space, or are you going to concede? The inertia of Flight makes excuses and never commits because it is never the right time and they are never quite ready. My decree to flighters is to buckle up buttercup: step up or shut up.

Flight is like minimum security prison, where you get little privileges, like walking the yard or reading a book. Freeze, on the other hand, is solitary confinement. To escape from your cell, you must look your jailers in the eye and prove that you are safe to the public. You, and you alone, must claim your freedom, because no one else can. There's an image of a bird sitting in a cage with the door open. Why does the bird stay in the cage? The victim voice keeps you safe in your little cage, your little bubble. If you are satisfied with this, then don't resent your circumstances and feel like a victim because it is your choice to stay small. I hope you eventually grow dissatisfied with this stagnant, small, status quo. The part of you that wants to grow inspires you to expand your perimeter and claim more space. Exploration is a righteous reason to push your boundaries, whereas if you are pushing back against the constraints, you will tend to get violent. If your Sensory Warrior is not intact, fighting for your rights gets ugly.

**Fight** injures others directly by attacking. This violation is obvious because it is overt and external. However, there is also a high internal cost to acting out against others. Malice erodes kindness and love is muted by hate. When we look at where these harsh feelings come from, we find a victim who didn't yet find their Sensory Warrior. Underneath the anger, there is grief. If you are unwilling to feel pain, it festers inside of you, and you will tend to inflict pain. This takes us back to false detachment, which is just an attempt to not Feel. If you *try* to let go, you aren't Releasing, you are Fighting. Fighters have to go back and Accept what happened and then Feel it. Once you Feel, you attach to what happened because it becomes personal when your entire body experienced it. It's now in you and part of you. It affected you and changed you deeply. How can you possibly Release it? It's not easy.

By the same token, how can you hold onto it? It happened and it is gone. If you want to re-litigate what was, you are out of touch with what is. If you stop your car on the freeway, you are resisting the flow and you might get rear-ended. The tough lesson here is that experiences pass through us. If we suffered, we might use that pain to define ourselves. Now that we identify with it, we are attached to it at the hip and we drag it around with us into our NOW. When we hold onto positive or negative experiences, our lens is skewed, and we fail to see the absolute value. We are still linked to what was, whether we hate or love it. If you resist pain, you'll get hardened and locked in an oppositional posture. Chronic pain is horrible, and no-one can judge resisting it. When you do actually Feel pain, and you manage to Release it, you have more compassion because you appreciate what suffering is. You wouldn't wish that on your worst enemy! Once you step back and look around, you might find that anyone you thought of as an enemy is just a poor fool who doesn't really know what they are doing. This isn't an excuse but rather a fact of life. Most people and animals are not particularly evolved yet, so we do things that hurt others, inadvertently or intentionally inflicting harm.

It's interesting that Flight needs to commit, and Fight needs to stop being so committed. This exaggerated commitment shows up as believing you are right, which is a slippery slope toward righteous indignation. Revenge, grievance, and retribution are also part of this persona. Vindicating yourself makes you vindictive. Your conviction fuels your Inner Prosecutor who wants to convict your Inner Defendant. This is when the Fight response creeps in and diverts your rightful thirst for your own space toward offense. If you don't get derailed here, your fierce energy empowers your Sensory Warrior that is devoted, discipled, and on the front line. Your Reboot Camp basic training opened your sensory side. The Intrinsic Breath introduced you to your Inner Witness, the one watching your body breathe all by itself. You learned that relaxing is a trust fall, and Free Fall took you airborne for paratrooper special ops. Self-healing awakens your parasympathetic Inner Healer, who catches your wounds. Now your Fight response gets reimagined into your Sensory Warrior who Accepts what is, Feels it and embodies it, and Releases what was.

A Sensory Warrior is a more interesting character than a savage fighter. Raw energy is vital, but when it's misguided, it causes harm. The anxiety of the Freeze response is a clear example of how detrimental adrenal energy can be when it gets shunted to the mind in an unbridled way. Raw rage has also ravaged and injured many innocent animals among us. However, when you tame this fire-breathing, adrenal dragon, you harness the raw power of your survival impulse. This forges a cadet into a warrior, and gives the Inner Protector martial artistry. Find your center and access your will, to fight the good fight, for a purpose greater than your Ego.

Claiming your personal space is a turf war. If someone yells at you, and pushes you back, how is your bubble going to respond? If someone asks you for your attention and energy, they are pulling you toward them. The front line is the membrane between your personal-space balloon and theirs. You supply the pressure, so you can either meet the moment, retreat, or implode. Fighters compensate for a previous implosion by exploding. True to yin/yang and Newton, the energy projected outwardly will be exactly equal, albeit opposite, to the amount they caved in. I said fighters are sheep in wolf's clothing, because the more they identify as a victim, the more zealous they get. Your Sensory Warrior is grounded and knows their power. They Feel when the bubble is neutral, so they don't overreact.

To recap, you started out imploded and frozen. Your Inner Protector repaired your boundaries and mended the membrane of your personal-space bubble. You stopped leaking Qi, re-inflated yourself, and gained ground. Once you find your personal equilibrium you can stop inflating yourself and just occupy your natural space. Be you, and stop trying to be more than that. Most of us don't even know our neutral self because we have been reacting to things our entire life. All of that EmoThinking and neural static makes it hard to just be your authentic self. You have to sneak up and stalk your Intrinsic Breath because the adrenal mind is so quick to judge. Asking yourself this simple question, "Who am I?" helps you drill down past the Ego's noise to reveal your intrinsic self.

In the Healing Your TimeLine segment I talked about converting an experience into a lesson, and I said that not every lesson is simple and neatly wrapped up with a bow on top. Your intrinsic self is an ever-changing mystery, and it is very slippery, so do not get too attached when you touch it. Your Sensory Warrior keeps applying and reapplying the Principles, staying with the flow.

**Fighting your own Breath**

The Corset and the Collar tells the story of toxic judgments. Taking a deep breath because you judge your breath as shallow seems innocent enough, but the subtext isn't so pretty. The EmoThinking mind created the background tension and put the corset and the collar on the body. Then the mind mindfully notices the breath and assesses it as shallow. At this moment the mind "should" offer a full apology to the body for creating the constriction. The mind could ask the body for forgivingness. To atone for its transgression; the mind could offer an act of service to regain integrity after causing harm. This rarely happens, but I invite you to try it.

Often, judgment creeps in, and the mind's mindful assessment gets weaponized against the body. The mind says, "You stupid body, don't you know anything? You suck at breathing. Do I have to everything around here?!?!" Your mind's reaction is to use technique to force the body to breathe better. Instead of removing the background tension, the mind whips the dumb beast so it performs parlor tricks. It's like a dystopian dog show where the owner makes the dog jump through a flaming hoop in order to be affirmed as being worthy. Aren't you worthy anyway, whether or not you take abuse and then blindly follow instructions? If you are litigating your worth, doubting your intrinsic value, and busy proving yourself, you aren't focused on self-healing.

How can you change this sad saga? Advocate, and appeal to the conscience of the abuser. Use your fighting spirit to advocate for yourself. If you are anxious, your body is suffering, and your mind is actively causing it. The mind can dish it out but it can't take it. Becoming a Sensory Warrior trains the mind to process moments cleanly, so the mind doesn't glom on to every experience and use that to define itself. Detachment challenges the adrenal mind to step aside so the parasympathetic side can stay present and cleanly process *what is.*

The ethic of Release can be enacted in several ways. Sometimes, tears are part of letting go, like the bittersweet sadness of saying goodbye to a loved one. Sometimes, a somber silence reflects the ennui of detachment. Other times, Release is expressed through laughter. Humor is the collision between yin and yang, when two opposing perspectives smash into each other and create a catharsis. These jokes don't shame the characters, they just help us see beyond our local perspective. Stop saying "bad monkey" to your body!! It's not nice!! This is serious business, but I invite you to retain your sense of humor when you dare to thaw out your buried content and Feel it. Sometimes, if you make fun of yourself, you let go of being so tightly attached to that part of you. That bird in the cage with the open door finally flies out when it stops being so serious and dares to let go and live a little.

# Identity Politics

We call humans social creatures, but that's just a fancy way to say pack animals. A tribe is a pack, complete with a code of conduct and a hierarchy, which is a pecking order. Groups often have strict roles, so if you break the rules, you get excommunicated or executed, shunned or stoned to death. In our modern culture, the law of the jungle becomes the law of the concrete jungle, and your survival depends on your place in the pecking order. For animals living in the wild, better eyesight, acute hearing, a thicker coat, or sharper claws make all the difference between life and death. For us, our social network and our financial capital are the big two assets that keep us alive. It boils down to money and friends. If you have money, you can buy shelter, food, and services like healthcare. The other major asset involves your allies and friends, people who empathize and are *simpatico*. If people like you, they will help you for free. Whether you pay with cash or you barter, you get what you need. Without money, you can't pay rent. Without friends, you are out of luck, and all alone in the world.

## Social Security

Friends make us safer and there is strength in numbers. If you are likable, it's easier to have friends. If you're grouchy, it's harder for your friends to be open. They might help you because they feel obliged, but they won't volunteer their resources as eagerly. It's funny to realize that being likable is a survival skill. When FaceBook hit the scene years ago, people were so eager to create their digital persona and show the world an idealized version of themself. I see this as an adrenal need to be accepted and affirmed, so that they don't feel alone in the world. Having FaceBook friends affirms their identity, which secures their place in the pecking order. Now I view the Ego, which governs the personality, as nothing more than an adrenal survival mechanism. We all depend and rely on each other, but when we desperately need friends to give us meaning, we fall into superficial bonds that don't satisfy our yearning for real intimacy.

As an experiment, look at your social motivations through this lens of survival. Notice any BelievEmoThoughts and apply the Principles to them. Your parasympathetic side wants to connect deeply. If you always act on your adrenal impulses, you end up isolating yourself and feeling lonely, even when you are with people.

**Financial Security**

Money motivates people because without money, we are vulnerable. People spend 40 hours a week or more working so they can get paid, and pay their bills. For many of us, the bulk of our time and energy goes into surviving. Even if you make enough money to pay for your needs, you might still be driven to make more money so you can have nicer things, vacations, etc. People can't seem to get off the hamster wheel and just be. Even many mega-rich folks tend to want more money and power because their adrenal ambition whispers in their ear that they aren't safe enough.

**Shunned or Stoned**

We don't bite each other in the carotid like wolves, but we incarcerate and execute criminals. Our version of shunning a member of our tribe is illustrated by how we collectively neglect poor people. Most people Freeze up and ignore a homeless person as they walk by, because they don't want to Accept that there is a person nearby who is in bad condition. It's easier to ignore them rather than face the fact. Part of the calculation to willfully ignore something or someone is to avoid being compelled to do something. Seeing is a commitment to being in reality, but you don't have to fix it. You can just acknowledge the reality you are in. When you walk past an unsheltered person, you don't have to save them, you can just say "hi" or nod to acknowledge that they exist. Like the Stenographer that only hears and doesn't Feel, you can Accept that this person exists, and continue along your way. You aren't guilty if you recognize they are there, even though it is difficult to see someone in rough shape. If you forgive yourself for having more than them, your heart will open and you might be able to genuinely help them. If you Freeze, you're actively shunning them.

## The Karmic Courtroom of Appeals:  Double Jeopardy

Water Under the Bridge sets up the courtroom where opponents litigate. If you lose in court, you can appeal to a higher court and re-litigate the case. It's interesting to point out that in the appeals court, the roles switch. The prosecution that won becomes the defendant in the appellate court. The original defendant who lost the case becomes the plaintiff who prosecutes their grievance in the appeals court. This role reversal demonstrates how defendants become prosecutors and how victims become perpetrators. It harkens back to passive-aggressive behavior and the transition from Flight to Fight.

Even more interesting is that your forgiving Judge doesn't rule on the case; they dismiss it and throw out the charges. Because there is no verdict, there is nothing to appeal, nothing to re-litigate. The legal term "double jeopardy" says that if you're accused of a crime and the case is dismissed, you can't be retried unless new evidence is presented. In this way, the dismissal is final and absolute, not relative and up for debate like a verdict. Dismissal doesn't just resolve the issue, it absolves you. You're not vindicated or castigated because your Inner Judge doesn't judge your adrenal characters. By seeing them all neutrally, they absorb the opposing charges, so they cancel each other out. By reconciling yin/yang, your Judge shows you your absolute value.

The appeals process of re-litigation continues the power struggle, which relates to karma and trading wounds. Adrenal survival programs endlessly litigate who's fault it is, and assign blame to the guilty party, the enemy, the other. Even fighting for your innocence occupies your energy and attention, wasting your precious Qi.

## Contract Disputes

If someone breaks a contract, they betray the agreement. The bond is broken, and the two connected parties are separated. It could be any real or perceived contract: a social interaction, a business venture, an oath, or a new year's resolution you make to yourself. Citizens are expected to follow the social contract of the tribe they belong to, which includes implicit rules of conduct and explicit laws. We can say that the person who breaks the contract is the offender or perpetrator and the person who didn't is the victim. People might be adversely affected, and the injured party can either forgive or not. If you break a vow to yourself, and you betray yourself, you become both the perpetrator and the victim. Interesting…

Forgiving someone doesn't mean you have to be their friend or trust them. It's just letting go of the old contract. You aren't giving your power to them or letting them take advantage of your kindness. When you forgive and *absolve* the old contract, there is no contract. You can make a new contract if you want, or you can decline to interact. The ball is in your court. Regaining control of your own narrative makes you safe, since safety =

control. If you suffered and lost energy by the betrayal, and you choose to Release it unconditionally, you are reclaiming your power back. Holding on keeps you stuck in an outdated arrangement, which wastes your Qi.

If you are holding onto the broken contract, and trying to enforce it in some way, then you are on the slippery slope of becoming the perpetrator in the relationship. Holding on becomes provocative, which is why Release is the remedy for Fight. Perhaps you want justice for being wronged, which sets you up to be vengeful, and willing to inflict harm. These thoughts can be, "I'll teach them a lesson!" The Biblical phrase of "an eye for an eye" is another occasion where Newton's "for every action there's an equal and opposite reaction" holds true. This is how yin/yang works and as the pendulum swings, victims become perpetrators and the cycle of violence continues through time. One reason this pattern can persist for so long is that many consider it fair to perpetrate harm once they *perceive* they were wronged. Maybe they were wronged and maybe they weren't, but if they feel justified in reflecting the damage, then everyone is indeed blind. Your eyes might work well, but when they are cloaked in judgmental darkness, there's no way they can see the light. Forgiving is a radical act.

## Clarifying Quantum Entanglements

Karma is crashed quantum entanglements and consciousness is clarified quantum entanglements. We generate consciousness by resolving yin/ yang and we generate karma by implementing the individual awareness that a yin or a yang perspective offers, which clearly has an opposite. If you identify as one side of yin or yang, you are buying into that local perspective, based on your circumstances and concept about what reality is. Quantum entanglement shows us that whatever spin a particle has, there's an antiparticle that has the opposite spin. When you believe you are an individual particle, you forget that you have a twin with the opposing spin. This is crashed because it ignores the fact that you and your mirror image are linked. If you believe in this false separation, that you are one of those particles and not both of them, then you only see one side of yin/yang.

This narrow viewpoint is karma. If you perpetrate harm, you will have to become the opposite spin side of that, which is the victim. Likewise, if you identify as a victim and you embody the victim energy, you're going to ultimately have to become the perpetrator to see the other side of what that is, which is the clarification of the quantum entanglement. This is what karma is for. It's not a bad thing. It's necessary so that you can resolve yin/yang, and you cannot resolve it falsely. You have to embody both sides completely to clarify the relationship between the opposing forces in order to find balance. When you hold both sides cleanly, you clarify your entanglements. This expands your awareness beyond your particle-self, because you recognize that you also have a distant twin that influences your spin. You and your shadow are inextricably tethered in a binary dance, a dualistic duet. Owning your entanglements enables you to detangle your attachments, and attain equanimity.

The Water Under the Bridge Meditation sets up the karmic courtroom with the accuser and the accused. Forgiveness is absolution, resolving the entanglement between Fight and Flight. Consciousness is generated from this process of seeing beyond your local perspective, while the karmic perspective limits you to reacting to your circumstances.

# Epilogue

As an experienced clinician, I recognize that every patient needs a precise remedy that's tailored to them. My treatments include manual therapy, acupuncture, herbs, and the words I say. Authors only have words. I can't assess you and give you my personal prescription that surgically identifies where you are stuck, but now you can identify the crashed loop you repeat. Some patients have metabolic issues that require additional molecules from foods, herbs, supplements, or medicines. Others have energy blocks. Physical ailments are issues with anatomical hardware and mental illnesses are glitches in neural software. Most patients, if not all, have a combination of metabolic and energy imbalance, so we need to address the entire system as a whole.

What I can do as an author is spell out the many aspects of your mind and body, so that you can find exactly what you need to know, hear, feel, experience, and process right now. Platitudes aren't precise and they miss the mark. Early chemotherapy was clumsy, because crude poisons kill all cells, not just the cancer cells. Distinguishing between healthy cells and malignant cells allows our medicine to target only the crashed cells. Refining our definition of self adds sophistication, whereas when the diagnosis is generic, the treatment is superficial.

When I introduced the 3 Principles, I said Accepting lets $x$ be $x$, so you let the sensations of this moment enter and come in. Feeling is processing the signals, giving you more decimal places that define your experience more precisely. Your Parasympathetic Inner Healer embodies these first 2 Principles. Deep empathy builds the awareness that keeps your self-image accurate and grounded in reality. Similarly, Einstein's Thought Experiments blended imagination with rigorous testing to shatter our old concepts and replace them with a better understanding. Every moment of mindfulness is an Experiential Experiment that researches truth.

As I wrote this book, I felt that every chapter was the most important chapter! While this seems impossible, I know that each individual reader needs to hear a particular message. I'll bet a dollar that at some stage in your life, when you're ready, you'll recognize this deep medicine too, in your own way. As a child, I was amazed by dandelions. These yellow flowers became white globes, seed pods that resembled spherical snowflakes. Just as kids blow out birthday candles to manifest their wishes, dandelion seeds drift in the wind in the hopes of finding fertile ground to sprout a new, living plant. There are many seeds embedded in these words, and there's fertile ground in you that wants your inner garden to grow.

Visit **www.PacificCenterOfHealth.com** for information about Adrian's clinic. Our excellent team of practitioners offers acupuncture, cupping, gua sha, herbal medicine, massage, cranial osteopathy, and Visceral Manipulation.

Visit **www.RebootYourNervousSystem.com** for more information, including audio meditations and a glossary of terms.

**Glossary**

**Reboot Website**

**Audio**

**Follow on Instagram**

Made in the USA
Monee, IL
29 January 2024

52077411R00129